Praise for

Heart Vision

"Dr. Dellia delves intensely into very core issues of societal shame, secrecy, self-denial and fear of judgement that imprison victims of abuse in years of pain with the potential of resultant intergenerational pain, anger and abuse.

I recommend *Heart Vision* to every man or woman who is struggling or knows someone who is struggling with the decision to end any type of abuse in their intimate relationship, with the understanding that the abuse can be physical, emotional, verbal, and/or financial.

Dr. Dellia encourages you (or one whom you care about) to recognize the RED FLAGS, confront the EVIL and have the courage to decide what you are going to do to retake control over your life."

—**RON LEGRAND, J.D.,** Attorney, Consultant and President and CEO of the LeGrand Group, LLC with expertise in policy and legislative affairs in the areas of gender-based violence, human trafficking, and criminal justice reform

HEART
VISION

HEART VISION

How to See Your Path Forward
When You're in a Dark Place

DR. DELLIA EVANS

ISBN 978-1-7341287-0-3 (print)
ISBN 978-1-7341287-1-0 (Kindle ebook)
ISBN 978-1-7341287-2-7 (ebook)

Cover and Interior Design by Jerry Dorris
Edited by Madalyn Stone

First Printing 2019
Butterflies Publishing
Jackson, MS 39236

For more information on buying this book in bulk, please
email visible@drdellia.com.

Printed in the United States of America

A Note from the Author

Everyone's relationship is different and should be addressed accordingly. What may work for one relationship may not work for another. The suggestions in this book are my personal opinions based on my personal experiences, so your experience may not be the same. Therefore, I cannot be responsible for your outcome. The information in this book does not take the place of going to a professional behavioral health therapist who can best advise you on your individual situation.

— Dr. Dellia Evans

Table of Contents

Foreword

Dr. Dellia candidly and boldly discusses the time in her life when she was in a dark place and ensnared by the sustained emotional, psychological, financial, verbal and eventual physical abuse in her marriage.

Her reasons for staying and the impact it had on her life and that of her children are the same as it is for many persons who are victims of Intimate Partner Violence (aka domestic violence). It is an unfortunate reality that we do not want to acknowledge that IPV exists. Another reality is that both men and women can be a victim of IPV.

When people began in a relationship the last thing that they believe will happen is that the person they think is great, kind, genuine, caring and loving turns out to be someone quite different. The man or woman of their dreams becomes the nightmare they could not imagine. What was once a beautiful relationship is now sinister and ugly.

I am a Licensed Professional Counselor (LPC) and Certified clinical Trauma Professional (CCTP) in a Christian counseling center and volunteer for IPV groups. I have had the opportunity to walk with numerous women and men on their journey of being or having been abused by their partners.

I have seen once thriving people reduced by the emotional, mental, spiritual, sexual and physical abuse into people who are afraid or don't believe they can make a simple decision.

Children in these situations are exposed to violence and

learn that the unhealthy relationship that they have seen is the way a relationship should be. They can then in turn become either perpetrators of or victims themselves of IPV.

With awareness of IPV, we can help and stop the intergenerational transmission (passing from one generation to next generation). This awareness can assure that homes are those of peace, respect, trust, genuine regard and love rather than homes of trauma.

I have also had the opportunity to work with teenagers and college students who are or have been in abusive relationships. One of the saddest cases I worked with was a child in middle school whose boyfriend hit, slapped and pinched her. Seeing a child who now has low self-esteem and a tainted view of relationships is heartbreaking.

The most frequent IPV questions of:

- "Why did he/she do this?"
- "How can they say they love me and treat me like this?"
- "What did I do to deserve this?" and
- "How can I make him/her stop?"

are ones that Dr. Dellia asked herself and are discussed in this book.

Victims of IPV try to be and do whatever their partner wants them to be until they get to the point where they lose themselves in the process. They are guided by fear of the abuser and what he or she will do to them and even their children, that they do whatever is demanded of them.

This book is a roadmap for those in — on their way out of — or are already out of IPV situations. This book is a must read for anyone who has been, is currently in or knows someone who is in an IPV relationship. To the latter group of people, we must help those who are in these situations and remove our blinders and preconceived thoughts.

I will recommend *Heart Vision* to **all applicable clients/ groups** because Dr. Dellia's story is one that anyone in IPV situations can relate and find strength.

Once blinded **they**–like Dr. Dellia–will be able to SEE (Spiritually Enlightened and Encouraged). They will learn that they have worth/value, deserve respect and dignity and have love...love that is authentic, uplifting, dynamic and free of shame, guilt and fear. This is the love we all hope to have and need. This is the love that God created us to have and share with others.

Stephanie Smith-Jefferson, MS, MA, LPC, CCTP
Assistant Director; Consultant/Counselor
Crossroads Counseling Center

Introduction

I'm an optometrist by profession. I've helped thousands of people to see more clearly. Because of my personal life's circumstances, however, I felt compelled to write *Heart Vision* to be a metaphorical light in the dark, to help survivors and victims of domestic violence see their paths forward from a dark place.

You can choose whether you'd like to read each chapter consecutively or pick and choose the chapters to read that interest you the most.

In *Heart Vision*, each chapter explains the meaning of each part of the acronym MAP to SEE. You can use this MAP as a guide so that you can SEE where you are on your journey, and then see how to move forward to your life's purpose.

The MAP to SEE acronym identifies six blind spots that could keep you from moving forward. One blind spot is revealed in each chapter. Once these areas of your life become visible, you will be able to move forward with more confidence. In each chapter, I recommend that you use a journal to record how to shine your light—how to look at your situation through the best lens to give you a higher perspective, focus on the big picture, and look with your heart.

It was my dad who first taught me how to look with my heart. You see, growing up, I was always Daddy's little girl. My dad was a simple janitor, but he was so wise and caring that everyone just loved him. He built us a 3,500-square-foot home in Jackson, Mississippi. We moved in when I was ten years old in 1978. I was thrilled because my bedroom was pink, just like I wanted.

I will never forget sitting on his lap, asking him, "How did you know how to build this house?"

He explained, "My spirit guided me. That is where God leads me from when I don't know what to do on my own. That is how I built this house. I never built a house before. I would ask God questions, and from a place deep inside, I would either hear His still small voice, or when I closed my eyes, He would show me in my spirit what to do with my hands and where to go with my feet."

I was still confused, so I asked, "What do you mean, your spirit?"

He went on to say, "Doctors know that in order for our bodies to stay alive, our heart has to keep beating to pump blood to it. Doctors know how to cut in the chest, where to find the heart, and how to repair damaged hearts. But they can't find the spirit. That is the real life of a person. The spirit of a person comes from God for a specific purpose when he or she is born. When we die, our bodies can't enter heaven, only our spirits. The spirit is invisible to man, but God can see it. That's where He communicates to us and shows us what to do. That's our spiritual heart."

I slid off my dad's lap, walked slowly down the long hallway back to my pretty pink room, and thought about what he had just told me.

Eight years later, when I went to college at Ole Miss, I could not see the screens in the large lecture rooms. My dad took me to the optometrist for the first time. I remember how my dad helped me pick out my first pair of eyeglasses. They were the least expensive and the ugliest ones in the optical shop. But when my eyeglasses were ready, and I put them on, I did not even think about their appearance. My eyes opened wide, and my mouth dropped open with gleeful surprise. I pointed and shouted, "Oh, my goodness! I can see the individual leaves on the trees!"

Before I put on eyeglasses, the leaves had only looked like green blobs. I thought they looked like that to everyone. For the first time, even though they had been right in front of my face the whole time, I saw everything that I had been missing clearly. That day, on my ride home from the optometrist's office, I said to myself, "I am going to do this for other people one day. I want to help other people see what they have been missing." That is why I became an eye doctor.

Fast-forward fifteen years...I was in Jackson, Mississippi working in an eye clinic. I was about to go into a patient's room to do an eye exam when I heard that still small voice on the inside say to me, "You are my optometrist."

I looked up at the ceiling and said under my breath, "What?"

The voice said, "You are the optometrist that I will use to not just help people see with their natural eyes. You are the optometrist that I will use to help people see with their spiritual eyes." I pondered that for a moment. I entered the exam room and finished examining my patient.

Five years later, I had to use my own spiritual eyes when I lost nearly everything—my marriage, house, car, job, and my life as I knew it. I had to flee the state of Oklahoma with my two young children after getting a restraining order and a divorce decree served to my husband.

I found myself back in the pink room of the house that my dad had built. I did not know what I was going to do.

I closed my eyes and asked God, "Show me in my spirit what I need to do with my hands, and where I need to go with my feet." In my spirit, I saw for the first time that my husband had not shown me the respect nor the love and security that I deserved; but most of all, I saw myself being happy.

For the next ten years, as I allowed my spirit to lead me; I found everything that I thought I had lost, and more. Today, I own a medical eye care practice and optical shop. While at work one day, one of my female employees came into my office, and she told me about her destructive relationship with her children's father.

She said, "I am so ashamed and tired of how he mistreats me and my children at home."

I shared my story with her. Then I said, "You deserve to be treated with love and respect." I gave her information about community resources that could help her. I said, "Close your eyes and see yourself and your children today. Now, deep in your heart, see how you all will look when you are free from your unhealthy relationship and resettled into a quiet and peaceful place." After more encouragement, my new, loving husband and I helped her follow her heart and safely leave her abusive home that very next Saturday.

As I thought about this employee, the more I realized how many women all over the world are struggling in similar situations. They are yearning for a brighter future. You may be one of these women. Because you may have been in the same place for so long, you may not see the reality of where you really are. You may not see how to move forward when you look around at your circumstances. My mission now is to help women just like you to not only see more clearly what you have been missing that has been right in front of your face but also to see a brighter future with the eyes of your heart.

Now you understand why I just had to write *Heart Vision*, because I've been there. I know what it's like to feel the craziness, disappointment, and the betrayal. I know what it takes to get to the other side of the fears and anxieties of a destructive marriage. I know what you need to do to find your way to a safe place of well-being and rest. And I want to help you get here.

By the time you have finished reading *Heart Vision*, you will learn what you can do to change your life. You will see the reality of your situation. You will discover what you have not been able to see that is keeping you stuck. Be true to yourself. Catch a clear vision in your heart of where you are going. And finally, be empowered to run with that vision.

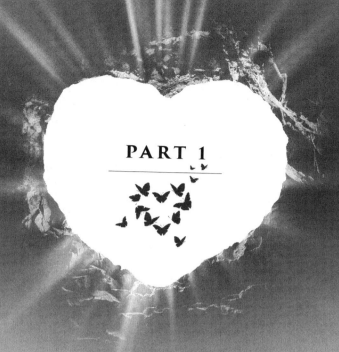

PART 1

M.A.P.

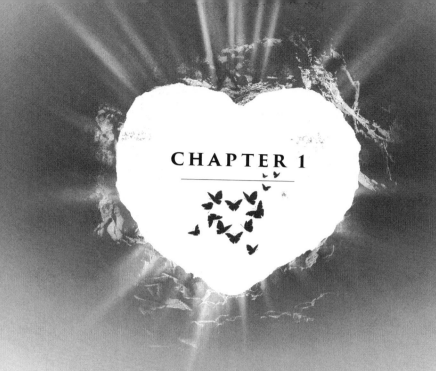

CHAPTER 1

M—Misinformation

MISINFORMATION CAUSES A MYOPIC VIEW

In the same way that you have blind spots in your natural eyes, you also have blind spots in your spiritual eyes. Each capital letter in the acronym MAP to SEE represents a blind spot that can figuratively keep you from seeing how you need to move forward with your life if you feel like you are stuck in an abusive marriage.

This metaphoric blind spot is different from the blind spot associated with driving a car. You see, your natural eye has a *blind spot*. There is a small space of your visual world that your eye does not see because there is an area in the back of your eye (called the *retina*) where there are no cells to receive visual information for that space. You do not notice that there is a missing space in your vision because your amazing brain "fills in" that space from the visual messages it receives from the other cells that surround the blind spot.

Have you ever given anyone "the thumbs-up?" You can find your blind spot in your right eye by doing the following exercise by using the thumbs-up sign: Go to the bathroom. Look in the mirror at your right eye. Close your left eye. Extend your right arm out in front of you. Make a fist and align your right thumb under the image of your right eye in the mirror. As you continue to look straight ahead at your right eye, very slowly move your thumb in a straight line to your right. Even though you are looking straight ahead at your right eye in the mirror, you will notice in your side vision that the tip of your thumb will disappear as you move your fist to the right. You have just found your blind spot in the right eye.

You have a blind spot in each eye. You can find the blind spot in your left eye, too. Just swap the words *left* for *right* and vice versa in the above exercise. You don't have to look in a mirror to find your blind spot. As long as you have one eye closed, and you look at a target straight ahead, and you slowly move something in a line out to that spot, you will find it. It has always been there, right in front of your face, and you did not even realize it.

In this chapter, you will be able to see how the first *blind spot of misinformation* can cause you to have a myopic or limited viewpoint. If you don't have a clear understanding, not only does it limit your perspective, it can also limit your behavior.

Myopia is a medical term that describes the condition of

being *nearsighted*. In this condition, you can only see objects clearly that are right in front of you. So, when you have a *myopic view*, you cannot see anything clearly that is at a distance from you. In other words, you cannot see the big picture.

If you are misinformed about your *free will*, God's opinion of divorce, what *biblical submission* really means, and honoring Christ, you will continue to stumble around because you can't see clearly to find your way out of the chaos of an abusive marriage.

MISINFORMATION ABOUT FREE WILL

Did you know that you (or other people who assist you) have to be the ones to perform the actions in your life because God does not run your life? Did you know that if you use your free will, you can receive God's promises? But for every promise God has for you, there is a condition attached to it.

Throughout scripture, you see that if you do this, then you shall have that. Even your very salvation works like this. God gives you the authority to make your own choices in life. He gives you free will. For God's sovereign plan to work in your life, you have to CHOOSE to do it. God exists outside of time. He can look at your past, present, and future all at once. He knows what choices you will make. Nothing sneaks up on Him and surprises Him. God said in the Bible that He puts life and death before you, blessings and curses. According to Deuteronomy 30:19, He tells you to CHOOSE life!

My marriage was dead. I had to decide with my own free will to CHOOSE life. For years, I thought that God would just miraculously change my situation for me if I just kept on fighting the good fight of faith. I thought that if I just stayed there and waited on the Lord, that He would somehow super-naturally show up and change things for me. Wrong! You are to pray and wait on God in your prayer time, but when you get up off of your knees, it's *your* responsibility to do something. You have to activate your faith to get manifestation in your life. For change to come in my and my children's lives, I had to be the one to make the decision to change and do something about it. I was the one that had to make the choice to leave. I asked myself, "Do you have faith in God, or not?" Faith without works is dead.

That horrible night when I made the choice to get a divorce, I knew I had to make a change. I had to make that choice for myself and my children to be safe and secure.

My son later told me, "That night, my fear caused me to stand there frozen as I watched Dad hurt you and my sister. I felt helpless."

What happened that night changed my life's trajectory.

Like me, as you put your faith into action, your change can happen step by step, as you allow God to direct your path. You have to believe that God will give you the courage to face your fears of: failure, the unknown, of possibly making the wrong move, losing everything that you have worked so hard to achieve, as well as the criticism of other Christians who are against the idea of divorce if you choose to do so. But remember, according to Deuteronomy 31:6, if you are strong and courageous, then God will be with you.

Did you know that your prayer of faith will not override the free will of others? For two decades, I stayed in a shattered marriage. I did not decide to leave my marriage because I was fasting and praying that God would change the heart of my husband.

The problem with that was that my prayers were coming up against the free will of what my husband wanted.

According to Mark 11:24, your prayers of faith work personally for you when they are in line with the Word of God. But according to Jeremiah 7:13-16, when another person's free will and faith are not in agreement with yours, those prayers are null and void, and God will not hear them.

I did try to get my vision in line with what I thought was God's vision. I tried talking and encouraging communication between me and my husband. For example, several months after I found out my husband had an affair, I arranged for us to participate in a Marriage Encounter–Marriage Retreat one weekend in April 2002. We went through all of the activities and the ceremony of renewing our vows, but after the weekend was over, his actions during the retreat did not line up with his actions that followed the retreat.

MISINFORMATION ABOUT GOD'S OPINION OF DIVORCE

Growing up going to church every Sunday and attending bible study during the week, I heard the message, "God hates divorce," many times. After getting married, I continued to hear this message being preached from the pulpit and in women's bible study. As a Christian woman wanting to do the right thing, I felt that divorce was not an option for me because I did not want to do something that God hates. Divorce must be a sin, right? The message was that unless your husband died or committed adultery, you were stuck. So, I stayed there in my marriage for twenty years.

When my husband committed adultery in January of 2002,

I had a way of escape. However, I never wanted to get a divorce. I was so nearsighted about trying to make my marriage work that I was not looking at the cost I was going to have to pay in the long run. I just focused on what I needed to do each day to keep my marriage and family together. I didn't want my children to grow up without their father. I wanted to fight for my marriage. However, by not leaving, I had decided to stay in my toxic environment.

I just believed that God would see me, hear my desperate prayers, and show up in the midst of my fire and rescue me. I found a Christian marriage counselor, and he assigned us a book to read called *Torn Asunder* by Dave Carder. This book offers hope, healing, and encouragement to couples who face adultery and want to move beyond it. I read this book through tears with the agony of a broken heart, asking God every night how I could ever trust again.

Asunder means to split apart or to separate. I held onto the scripture found in Mark 10:9 which says, "What God has joined together, let no man put asunder." What I misunderstood about this scripture was that any man or woman who continually disrespects and abuses his or her spouse has already torn asunder the relationship. *The spouse that is being abused is not the one that separates the relationship.*

This separation usually occurs in the privacy of one's home. A divorce is just an outward declaration to the public of what has already occurred days, months, or sometimes years before. So, if you make a decision to separate or divorce an abusive spouse so that you can be safe physically, financially, emotionally, and mentally, then you can move on to a more productive, fulfilling life knowing that this scripture does not apply to you.

I did not understand this at the time, so I continued to stumble around because of my nearsightedness.

When I went to church, I heard the message that "God hates divorce." It would usually come from the scripture reference Malachi 2:16, which says, "'I hate divorce,' says the Lord God of Israel, 'and the one who is guilty of violence,'" says the Lord who rules over all. "Pay attention to your conscience, and do not be *unfaithful*" (NET version).

Another interpretation of this same scripture says, "'Indeed, the Lord God of Israel says that He hates divorce, along with the one who conceals his violence by outward appearances,' says the Lord of the Heavenly Armies. So, guard yourselves carefully, and don't be *unfaithful*" (International Standard Version).

Yet another interpretation of this scripture says, "For the man who does not love his wife but divorces her, says the Lord, the God of Israel, covers his garment with violence, says the Lord of hosts. So, guard yourselves in your spirit, and do not be faithless" (English Standard Version).

As you continue to look at this scripture more closely, you can see that what God truly hates is the broken relationship caused by the husband not loving his wife and treating her cruelly. God does not like the husband rejecting his wife, putting her away, and treating her *treacherously or unfaithfully*. This is the type of relationship that God hates. We see all through the New Testament of the Bible that Jesus is more concerned about love and relationship than He is with trying to keep faith to every letter of the Mosaic law that the Pharisees and the Sadducees were trying to do. God does not want His daughter to live in this type of environment.

My godmother, Ms. Willa, who lives in Montgomery, Alabama had told me just that more than eight years before

I made the decision to leave my husband. I have known Ms. Willa since I was a little girl. I call her my godmother because she led me in a prayer of salvation to ask Christ to come into my heart when I was just nine years old. She also prayed with me to receive the power of the Holy Spirit to help me to be an effective witness.

I was overjoyed to reconnect with her as an adult after my family had moved to Montgomery. For two years, the first Saturday of each month, I would go to her house to help her prepare for a women's bible study that she held in her home. One particular Saturday in August of 2002, once again we had a wonderful time of fellowship with the ladies from church. Ms. Willa had shared her godly wisdom with us, and we ate delicious hors d'oeuvres that she had prepared as she always did. After I finished helping her clean up, and all of the other women had left, I was the last one there.

As I was about to leave, I turned to her as she said, "Dellia, I have been hearing some things about your husband from other people at church, and I am concerned about you." My heart sank. I did not know that anyone knew what I had been going through in my personal life. "I heard that he has not been keeping good company, and I don't want that to affect you."

Trying to save face, I reassured her that I was okay but that I did not know what she was talking about. Even though I knew my husband kept secrets about his life outside of our home, I honestly had not heard the details that Ms. Willa had just shared with me. But Ms. Willa saw right through my facade.

She continued, "God does not want His daughter to live a life of disrespect, hurt, pain, and mistreatment. God wants you to be free and delivered."

Then Ms. Willa's husband, Mr. Sam, chimed in, "Yes, Dellia, sometimes you have to just cut your losses."

Although that was the best godly counsel I could have received, at that time in my journey I was not at the point to receive it. I was totally in denial. I was looking at my situation from a myopic lens and just saw it as a bad patch in my marriage. We had just been to our marriage retreat four months before this conversation, and I was still hopeful. I did not see the true reality of it all. I was just trying to hold things together and get through each day. *Sometimes outsiders can see your situation more clearly from a distance than you can when you are succumbing to your circumstances.*

MISINFORMATION ABOUT BIBLICAL SUBMISSION

Just as I had heard many messages in church about God hating divorce, I had also heard a lot of messages about wives being submissive to their husbands. The message usually comes from Ephesians 5:22 and 24. Ephesians 5:22 says, "Wives, submit yourselves to your husbands as to the Lord" (Good News Translation). Ephesians 5:24 says, "And so wives must submit themselves completely to their husbands just as the church submits itself to Christ" (Good News Translation).

Many people reference wives submitting to their husbands from the scriptural excerpt where Paul is comparing the husband–wife relationship to that of Christ's relationship to the Church. But Christ's relationship to the Church is in no way violent, abusive, and disrespectful. That's why this comparison does not apply to any relationship that has these elements in it.

This message from Paul begins by saying there should be mutual respect between you and your husband. In a healthy relationship, both you and your husband would submit to the wishes of each other. You should both want the best for each other. Ephesians 5:21 says, "Submit yourselves to one another because of your reverence to Christ" (Good News Translation).

In the rest of this passage, Paul goes on to instruct husbands how to treat their wives—your husband should love, serve, and even sacrifice himself for you, if it is necessary, just as Christ did for the Church. This leaves no room for him to abuse you in any way. God does not want you to stay in harm's way and submit to your husband if he is treating you like a doormat.

Submission means to agree. We *submit* to God's will when we *agree* to the Word of God. When a husband submits or agrees with God, then his wife can submit and agree with him. That's what Ephesians 5:22 means, that wives should agree with their husbands as their husbands agree with God. If your husband is not in agreement with God, how can you be in agreement with him and bring glory to God?

The night after I made the decision to get a divorce, I remember crying and praying to God. I asked Him, "Why did You allow me to go through all of this if You knew this was going to happen?"

I heard His still small voice in my spirit say, "You had to find out for yourself. Now you see that you were not in control. If (my husband's name) didn't listen to Me, how do you think he was going to listen to you?"

You can substitute the words "agree with" or "submit to" for "listen to." I thank God for showing this to me in my spirit...in my heart vision.

Let's rewind back six and a half years. That would put us at five months after Ms. Willa and Mr. Sam had given me their wise advice. Since the time of their advice, things had gone from bad to worse in my marriage. I had been married thirteen years at that time.

In the following situation that I am about to tell you about, I knew that I could not be the submissive wife to my husband. I knew that according to the Bible; I was supposed to submit to my husband *as unto the Lord*. But when he asked me to do something that was not *as unto the Lord*, I knew that scripture did not apply.

It was January of 2003; the heart-wrenching marriage counseling after my husband's infidelity had not worked. In fact, my husband told me that he was leaving me and our children for "the other woman."

For several years, he had not been working or contributing in any way financially to the family household. He had made it a habit of making large withdrawals from our joint bank account several times a week although he was not depositing any money into it. So, I put a block on the checking account.

He was beside himself with anger, demanding, "Dellia, I need money to move to Florida." Of course, I said no. All of a sudden, he put a gun to my face. "Get me the money!" he snarled.

I was so tired of his antics that I told him, "Go ahead and shoot me. Send me to Jesus. You still will not have the money, and you will need to take care of the children."

Well, he obviously did not want to do that because he did not pull the trigger. Instead, he threw a tantrum. He started yelling, smashing things, slamming doors, and turning over things as he stormed out of the house. I called the police to make a report and they confiscated the gun. The next morning, he came and dropped the children off at school. Instead of going to work, I went to the school and withdrew our children. I went to the bank and withdrew the money and got on the interstate heading to Jackson, Mississippi four hours away.

He found out that I did not go to work that day. He went by our children's school and found out that I had checked them out. He called my parents whom I had told I was coming. For some reason, they told him that I was on my way there. I had not told them any details. He got in his car and began a hot pursuit of me and our children.

He called multiple times like a mad person ranting and raving, leaving an alarming number of threatening messages. When I got to my parents' house, I told them that I could not stay there because it was too dangerous. I told them that I had left without packing a thing. They went by a Dollar Store and picked up some toiletries and a basic change of clothes for me and their grandchildren.

I told them that my husband was about an hour behind me on my tail and that I was going on to his parents' house another two hours north. I thought I would be safer there. I did not tell my parents any details. I'm sure they knew I was desperate. My parents volunteered to drive us there. I passed out on the backseat on the way there from the exhaustion of my "fight and flight" response.

A year before this happened, I had packed a suitcase for myself and for my children and left my husband when I could not bear the pain of a broken heart because of the betrayal of his infidelity. After he found out that I was gone, he coaxed me to come back with his convincing apologies and promises.

This time was different. I felt as if I were prey being hunted down by a predator. I felt as if I were trying to escape with my life. I knew deep down inside that I needed to make a change. But the cycle of abuse continued after he finally caught up with me. More apologies and promises followed. We went to talk to a preacher that my husband knew who was a friend of his family. I was again entangled in the web of misinformation.

I refused to go back to Alabama. I had no support system there. I stayed in Mississippi, and my husband eventually moved there to join us. He started attending Word of Faith Christian Center in Jackson where I had become a member. He went to the alter and repented before the church and God. I wanted to believe him. I was still quite nearsighted. On our wedding anniversary in August of 2003, the assistant pastor renewed our wedding vows once again. Unfortunately, after a few months, the same destructive behavioral patterns emerged. I did not tell anyone my secret. I continued to believe that God was going to work a miracle in my husband. I stayed in my destructive marriage six more years. But my marriage was not reflecting the image of Christ's love for the Church.

MISINFORMATION ABOUT HONORING CHRIST

I challenge you to focus on what truly honoring Christ really means. You can be honoring your own vision and not be honoring Christ. With my myopic view, I thought I was honoring Christ by staying in a bad marriage. I really wasn't. I was only honoring my own vision of staying married at all cost. *In reality, when you are in a marriage where you are continually being mistreated, that is not honoring Christ or giving God any glory.*

You know that your life is honoring Christ because of the fruit that it bears. If the reality of whatever vision you are running with is not taking you to a place where you are bearing spiritual fruit, your vision is not of God. Your vision is not lined up with God's vision. And you will not be in the place where He wants you. You will be in the wilderness of your life.

For twenty years, I was going around and around in circles, not getting anywhere, just like the children of Israel, until one horrible night. That was the night when I saw how the emotional trauma of my abusive marriage with their father was affecting my children, and then I knew that staying in my marriage was not honoring Christ.

The Holy Spirit finally got my attention, and that caused be to move forward toward my place of rest. God's vision and plan for your life will always be in a place where spiritual fruit is being produced and experienced. The fruit of the Spirit is love, peace, joy, kindness, gentleness, patience, goodness, faithfulness, and moderation.

Even though you may be offering these character traits, you may not be on the receiving end in a bad marriage. I wasn't. Quite the opposite; spoiled fruit was being produced instead. That's how you know when your marriage is not honoring Christ.

One example of the spoiled fruit that was being produced in my life occurred one month before I decided to get a divorce. It was in June of 2009. My family was living in Tulsa, Oklahoma at the time. On this particular morning, I refused to give my husband some money because I needed it for household bills. He was not helping me pay these bills, and he would not tell me what he needed the money for. I came home that Wednesday evening with my mind on getting ready to go to bible study at Rhema Bible Church with my children. But I did not make it that night.

When I walked into my bedroom, it looked like we had had a break-in from someone looking for money. The room and my closet had been ramshackled. All my dresser drawers had been pulled out. My clothes were everywhere. Many of my things were broken, other personal items had been tossed around in disarray. I remember picking up a broken picture frame with our wedding photo in it. The glass in front of the photo was cracked and shattered.

Sweeping up the chips of glass was a foreshadowing of my cleaning up the broken pieces of my marriage and life one month later. In July of 2009, I finally decided to use my free will and make a decision to get a divorce. Before then, I was not experiencing any of the fruit of the Spirit...I only cried and choked on "sour grapes." That Wednesday night, I just tried my best to put everything back in place and go back to my life as usual, but I never could.

Are you trying to put the broken pieces of your marriage and your life back together but finding that you can't put it all back together again? Is your husband unfaithful to you? Do you see how your marriage is not honoring Christ and not bringing God glory? Are you submitting (or agreeing) with your husband, but he is not submitting (and agreeing) with God? Are you so focused on keeping your marriage vows in a destructive marriage that you are not looking at the big picture of how it is affecting you and your children in the long run?

If you answered yes to any of these questions, you may have just located yourself on this MAP to SEE that you need to exercise your free will and make a decision to change your life for your sake as well as for that of your children.

YOUR DIVINE REFLECTION

The Best Lens

In your journal, write down the best lens (or scriptures) to look through in the Word of God so that you will not have myopic vision because of misinformation.

Here are three examples to get you started:

1. "Wisdom is of utmost importance, therefore get wisdom, and with all your effort work to acquire understanding." Proverbs 4:7. International Standard Version
2. "If any of you lacks wisdom, you should ask God, who gives generously to all without fault, and it will be given to you." James 1:5. New International Version.
3. "This day I call the heavens and the earth as witnesses against you that I have set before you, life and death, blessings and curses. Now choose life, so that you and your children may live." Deuteronomy 30:19 New International Version

The Big Picture

In your journal, write your own prayer to God that He will give you His eternal view and that you will not be limited by the nearsightedness of limited understanding.

Here is my prayer for you:

Father God, You are all-knowing and full of wisdom. Thank You for giving my sister Your wisdom and understanding for what You would have her to do in her life concerning her marriage. Give her Your viewpoint on how her choices are affecting her now and, in the future, and how they are affecting other people in her life. Help her to realize what a healthy relationship looks like. Lead her to a place where she can enjoy giving and receiving the fruit of the Spirit every day. Let her only agree with those who are in line with Your will. Help her to choose what brings life to her on every level of her well-being—spiritually, physically, emotionally, and financially. In Jesus' name I pray. Amen.

Heart Vision

Close your eyes and look with your heart at what your life looks like now and what you want your life to look like three months, six months, one year, and five years from now. When you open your eyes, write in your journal what you saw.

Answer these questions in your journal:

- Are you being treated like God wants His daughter to be treated? If not, are you exhausted and tired of being treated like you are? Describe how you are being treated, and how that makes you feel.
- Are you agreeing to requests that are not as the Lord would desire? If yes, how?
- Is your marriage honoring Christ and giving God glory? If not, what are the fruits that your marriage is producing if they are not the fruit of the Spirit?
- In your heart, what do you want for your marriage, your children, and your home?
- If God's will for your life is different from yours, are you open to accepting that? If you are open, how can accepting God's will be better for you? If not, why are you not open?

Shining Your Light

Hopefully, you no longer have the blind spot of misinformation discussed in this chapter that some women might have.

In your journal, write three things you can do this week to let your light shine and to put your heart vision into motion. Answer these questions in your journal:

- If you are being abused in your marriage, what choice will your make to cause a positive change in your life?
- What can you do to truly honor Christ when it comes to your marriage?
- Who can you make an appointment with to get godly counsel if you are not being treated as God's daughter should be?

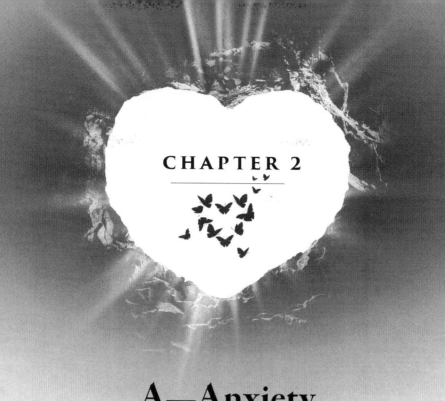

CHAPTER 2

A—Anxiety

ANXIETY CREATES PANIC AND CLOUDS YOUR SIGHT

"**A**m I going to need a Seeing Eye dog?" is what one of my patients frantically asked me when I told her that she had glaucoma several years ago. She started sweating, breathing hard, and rocking back and forth in the exam chair. Her eyes welled up with tears.

I handed her a Kleenex and said, "Oh, not at all. Just relax. Take a deep breath. Your condition is very mild. We have caught it early. We will work together to reduce your risk of future vision loss."

It was as if I had not said anything. Her voice went up an octave and started to tremble when she quickly rattled off, "I know that glaucoma causes blindness and that there is not a cure. If I go blind, I will not be able to get around. I will not be able to drive or work or pay my bills. I will not be able to function at home, or even see to myself, and I just know that my children will not take care of me."

I saw that she had become overwhelmed with emotion. At that moment, nothing else that I said about her diagnosis or treatment plan mattered. All that she could see in her heart was hopelessness and despair. She did not want to face her fear of the possibility of going blind from "The Silent Thief of Sight, Glaucoma."

She happened to be a member of my church, so I asked, "Is it alright if I pray with you?" She nodded her head yes. I reached out my hand, and she opened her clinched fist and took it. We closed our eyes, and I said a prayer of faith with her.

During the prayer, I said, "We thank You, God that You are in control, that You see us, and that You love us. We thank You that You are the Great Physician. We agree that You are still causing eyes to see both physically and spiritually. We agree that You are the same God yesterday, today, and forever." I closed the prayer, and we opened our eyes. Her whole countenance looked different. She was now calm and smiling. I finished counseling her about her treatment plan. She thanked me, and I left the exam room.

ANXIETY—INVISIBLE BUT REAL

That woman is still my patient. She is seeing well today. Her eye health has remained stable. As I think back on that day, I know that she was having a panic attack. Panic attacks are caused by overwhelming anxiety. Have you ever had one? Think about how you felt. What triggered it? Before it happened, did you realize that the trigger was causing that much stress? Sometimes you are not aware of how much stress you have or its impact on you. Anxiety is the second blind spot of the acronym MAP to SEE that we talk about in this chapter. It is invisible, but its effects are real.

Anxiety and fear can be present under the surface all the time, but you may not even realize that they are the reasons you feel stuck. Anxiety can be the blind spot that leaves you feeling paralyzed and unable to move forward. *Subconsciously, anxiety from your thoughts of worry and dread and stress can take such a toll on you that it results in an emotional response that manifests in your body, which then tries to shut down as a default coping mechanism.*

MY PANIC ATTACK

I did not realize the amount of anxiety that I had until I experienced the symptoms of a panic attack myself. I remember the day that I was at the circuit clerk's office in Tulsa, Oklahoma in July of 2009. The woman at the booth said, "Just sign here." It was the paperwork for a restraining order on my husband to protect me and my children. I just stood there staring at the paper.

I could not believe this was happening to me. At that moment, I was petrified by the fear of the unknown and what my husband would do to me because of this decision. I wondered, "Would he react to this restraining order by increasing his threats or physical violence against me and the children?"

Time seemed to stand still. I felt sick in the pit of my stomach. I started getting hot and clammy and hyperventilating. I got weak in the knees, and my feet felt like I was standing in two blocks of cement. I could not move.

The clerk said to me, "Calm down. You can do this."

I shook my head and whispered, "No, I can't do it."

She said, "Think of your children."

From my spirit came the scripture, "I can do all things through Christ that strengthens me." I closed my eyes and took a deep breath. I slowly let it out. *All I could see in my heart was the fear in my two children's eyes from three nights before as they watched their dad go into an uncontrolled rage and later told me that they did not want to stay in the place where they called home anymore.* I opened my eyes. My vision had been cloudy, but now it was clear. I signed the paper and walked out of the office feeling numb.

MY PERSONAL STORY

Until now, I have only made references to the events that took place just three nights before I signed those papers. That night marks the turning point of my life. Before I share my personal story with you about that night, I first want you to know that I believe in miracles.

For twenty years, I prayed and held onto the belief that God was going to save my marriage. After all, isn't that what we do as Christian women? Pray that God will intervene in our dysfunctional relationships? The truth is, I wasn't ready. I wasn't prepared. I was busy being a godly woman. At the time that meant that I protected my vows even though I was abused, betrayed, and ended up broke and broken.

Throughout those two decades, I received countless signs that my children's and my mental, emotional, physical, and financial well-being were at risk. But I kept praying and waiting for God to create the vision that I held for my marriage. I wanted to see that vision fulfilled. That was my prayer to God. Regardless of what was happening or what God was showing me, my idea of what my marriage could become was my daily focus and fight. And that's where I stayed until July 2, 2009.

My family was living in Tulsa at the time. It was an early morning, about 1:00 a.m. I was lying in the dark, wide awake. I was once again waiting for my husband to come home. I turned over in the bed and waited. I could hear him insert the key into the lock and turn it. I suspected he was out with someone else—again. It had happened so many times before I couldn't even be angry anymore. But I was still frustrated, disappointed, and hurt.

My husband entered our bedroom. He turned the light on. I asked, "Where have you been?" Of course, he made up a fictitious story; in other words, he lied. I turned over in the bed and started praying. As usual, he started antagonizing me. He wanted to justify his behavior by provoking a negative response. I decided to wait on God. It wasn't long after that a physical altercation ensued, and my children were awakened by the chaos. They witnessed the violence. They became the victims of my husband's and my unwise choices.

That night was my turning point. The police arrived and arrested my husband. For my safety and the safety of my children, the officer advised me to leave our home as soon as possible. He gave me a card so that I could contact a shelter for battered women. After the police took my husband and headed for the police station, I came to myself. In shock and shame, I looked in my young children's eyes and saw their terror. That is when my daughter said, "I don't want to be here anymore." My son said, "I want to go to Grandma's house in Jackson." At that point, I knew they needed my protection, love, and courage.

That's when I decided that it was over. God didn't have to wait for me any longer. *I thought that I had been waiting on God. But all the time, He had been waiting on me.* He was waiting on me to use my free will and take action, to step out on faith and believe that He loved me and wanted a better life for me. He wanted me to believe that He would take care of me and my children. Well, that night, I was ready. I made the decision: I was going to leave my husband for good this time.

I told my children to pack an overnight bag, and I did the same. We left to find a secret, safe place to hide. We found refuge in an express hotel about thirty miles away. At daylight, I went to my attorney's office and filed for a divorce. I then drove my children to the safest place I knew—my parents' home.

That ten-hour drive to Jackson, Mississippi gave me plenty of time to think, pray, and ask questions—questions that I didn't have all the answers to. But I knew this: My vision for my ideal marriage with my then husband was shattered, but God's purpose for my life was born.

Two days later, I drove back alone to Tulsa and stayed temporarily to complete more legal and work obligations. One of those matters was getting the restraining order. A couple of hours before I had the panic attack in the circuit court's office, I had to present my case in front of a judge.

The judge asked me, "Why are you here?" I started telling him about the events that had recently occurred. I told him that I drove my children to my parents' house over the weekend for their safety. I told him about our previous history of abuse in Alabama, how I felt because of the harassing phone calls, and how I was afraid to go back to the house to stay.

At that moment, images from my entire marriage flashed in front of my face. In front of the courtroom, right then and there in front of the judge, I burst out and started crying hysterically. I don't remember what happened next, only that I ended up in the office of a chaplain of the court. The next thing I remember is standing in front of the circuit clerk.

Throughout the next two weeks, I met with my boss and had more visits with my attorney. It became apparent that I had to leave permanently, quicker than expected because my husband was stalking me and not adhering to the restraining order. I abruptly left the state upon the advice of my attorney.

I was bound for a new place, a new life, and new opportunities. I didn't know exactly what or where. As I headed back toward my parents' house once again, it was clear my marriage and the life that I knew was over—really over this time. I now had another prayer, "God, what do I do next?"

Fear is a God-given emotion that tells you that there is a threat. Fear tells you that you need to get out of danger. My children and I were in a dangerous situation. We had to get to a peaceful place of security, safety, and rest. All throughout my journey, no matter how things looked, I would always recite Isaiah 32:18. It says, "My people will live in peaceful dwelling places, in secure homes, in undisturbed places of rest." Whenever there was confusion, I would recite this scripture to my children and husband. Today, this scripture has truly manifested in my life. I had a plaque made with this scripture on it. It is hanging up in the foyer of my present home.

When your fear turns into anxiety and worry and stress that paralyzes you, you can find protection and relief if you ask God to help you deal with it and move on. Moving on is the key. According to I Peter 5:7, you should, "Cast your anxieties on Him, because He cares for you."

THE FEAR OF FAILURE

I have a round, orange pot pad in my kitchen that I have had for years. I have never used it for getting hot items out of the stove or microwave because I use it as a decoration on my wall. It says, "ROUND TUIT — How many times have you said, 'I'll do it as soon as I get around to it?' Now's your chance. Now you can do it. Now at last, you've got A ROUND TUIT." Initially, I got the pot pad because I just thought it was cute.

I tend to procrastinate. Instead of putting things off, saying that I will get around to it, when I look at this pot pad I smile and say, "I already have gotten A ROUND TUIT." By eliminating that excuse, I get started sooner. I did not realize that I put things off because I had the fear of failure. This anxiety was a blind spot that has always been there, keeping me from moving forward.

Do you know of someone who is a perfectionist? I have been told that I am one. When you are a perfectionist, you want things to be done right. You want everything to fall in line right down to the smallest detail. I must agree that I have this tendency. I think I got it from both of my parents.

I remember my mother telling me, "Either you do it right, or don't do it at all." It's all or nothing if you are a perfectionist. You have a spirit of excellence. In church, I could relate to the song, "Ninety-Nine and a Half Won't Do." I remember as a child setting goals and achieving them. If I did not, I would either feel annoyed or devastated or blame myself too hard for failing.

One of the downsides of being a perfectionist is that you tend to procrastinate because you want to do things at the right time. You may procrastinate because: you are not ready to do something; because you feel you are not prepared enough; you are not doing something right; or everything else is not lining up just right. Because it is all about achieving your goal as a perfectionist, you tend to not care about what happens in between, what it takes to achieve it, and how long it takes. You sacrifice your time, energy, and resources at all cost.

This is exactly what happened in my abusive marriage. I had a fear of failure. Having a successful marriage was my goal. I wanted to see it through no matter how much I was hurting and disrespected. That is not God's will for your life.

Don't make the same mistake that I made. Don't keep trying desperately to make everything right all by yourself. If you are in a broken marriage, and you both are committed to working on it, it may be fixed. A destructive marriage is more than just broken; it is shattered. One person alone cannot simply put the pieces back together.

When you are in a marriage where there is continuous abuse and your partner refuses to change and care for your well-being, it is destructive. You are not in the type of healthy relationship that God desires for you to be in. Don't put off deciding to get help and putting a safe plan of action together if you are in a destructive marriage. If you feel that you are in physical danger, call 911. You can call a 1-800 hot line number for a professional advisor (see appendix B for resources). You are the one who has to make a choice of what to do and do it. (If you are not sure if you are being emotionally abused, take the quiz in appendix A to find out.)

Look in the Word of God to see what He wants for you. Pray for His wisdom on what to do. Ask for godly counsel from other Christians you trust and/or a professional Christian counseling center if possible. Look in your heart to see what you want. Then you have to take action. (We will talk more about how to do this in chapter 7 on "Moving Forward to Your Purpose.")

THE FEAR OF DISAPPROVAL

The Holy Spirit communicates with you differently than He communicates with me. Clearly, the Bible provides provisions for your mental, emotional, physical, and spiritual safety. Often, you may ignore these provisions because of your own internal challenges.

This I know for sure: Everyone has their reasons for their decisions. Sometimes, I wonder if not deciding to take action is as telling as not making a different decision. I believe you don't decide to take action because you don't want to make another mistake. You already feel and see yourself drowning and sense that any movement will only get you in deeper.

When you ask for advice, looking for answers about how to fix what's broken, you may only discover your situation is not just broken, it's shattered. The solution isn't about how to fix it, but how to abandon twenty, thirty, or forty years of your life—and that's scary.

You quietly wonder how making a change is going to interrupt your truth and everything else about your life. You know how things work now. You know where everything is—and isn't. And you have survived in this state. The thought of change brings into sight too many unknowns and questions. Will you go from bad to worse? Will you be left dangling in the air? You think, "Although what I have is dysfunctional, I have learned to work with it."

In the midst of my situation, I remember asking myself, how would I go from being married to being single? The thought of failing at marriage haunted me. I didn't want to accept the fact that I couldn't succeed at something I had set out to achieve. Of course, that was one of the many lies I was telling myself.

I had failed at other commitments. Why was this one so different? I surrounded my belief with this "truth" to justify my decision. Marriage is a sacred vow—a covenant among God, me, and my husband.

When one of my coaches asked me the following question, I had to admit that it was something different driving my behaviors. She asked me, "If no one knew you were married except God, your husband, and you, would you feel the same?"

I paused and uttered, "No!" I admitted to myself that it was more about the perception of others, especially my church family, than the commitment of marriage. I had been keeping up appearances for years. How could I explain what had been happening to other church members?

For years, I went to church and took my children every Sunday and midweek to bible study. Sometimes my husband went, and sometimes he didn't. We all looked good going to church. I acted like everything was normal. I had the same friendly smile and personality that I always had. I pretended that we were the ideal church family. I did not want anyone to know how awful things were.

I did not tell my church family, my biological family, my in-laws, or even my best friends. No one in my professional life knew. I was too embarrassed and ashamed of what was going on. I did not want to have any negative labels. As a woman of faith, I did not want to go against what I had been taught. So, I learned, to my detriment, how to dabble in my false hope rather than be rescued by a different, higher truth.

If I got a divorce, I thought the church people would shun me or look down on me. *I was held captive by the fear of disapproval. I was so concerned about the opinions of others that I did not reach out for help at the time when I needed it the most.* I don't want you to make the same mistake that I made. Find one or two godly people whom you trust, whom you can share what you are going through, who will listen, pray, and support you.

Again, while I was going through this part of my journey, I did not realize that this fear, these worries and concerns about others' opinions were keeping me bound, captive, immobile, and stuck in an abusive marriage. If you can identify this blind spot in your life, learn to get over other peoples' opinions. You should live your life for an audience of one. God's opinion is the only one that matters.

FINANCIAL WORRIES

When I first got married, I believed that my husband would always be there for our family spiritually, emotionally, and financially. My husband did take care of the finances for a while. I was not aware of his lack of financial management skills and his shopping addiction that led to thousands of dollars in credit card debt. I tried to help pay his debt down, but my efforts were to no avail because his spending was out of control.

When he was laid off from work, our daughter was three and our son was one year old. During the next thirteen years of our marriage, he did not contribute to the family's income in any consistent, meaningful way. He purchased vehicles in his name with money that I had earned without my knowing about it beforehand.

He was not contributing to the joint checking account, but he would overdraw the account by hundreds and hundreds of dollars consistently, and he would not tell me what it was for. *I went to an attorney concerning the past financial abuse. She said that she knew it was wrong, but legally nothing could be done because we were married.*

The last three years of our marriage, he worked full-time but still would not help me with any financial obligations. When I opened my own account to make sure that I could pay household expenses, he started to demand that I give him money even though he had just gotten paid. He got a car title loan from a loan shark and used fear to get me to pay it back. He got payday loans and overdrew credit cards that he did not pay back. I stopped answering the landline phone because of harassing debt collector's calls.

Money was missing from my purse, my closet, and the children's dresser drawers. There were always crazy stories about what happened to the money. One Christmas, he led me to believe that colleagues at work had stolen money out of my purse; it was money I needed to buy the children's presents. I even had the employees fingerprinted by the police. Looking back on it now, I realize that was a mistake. They were not the ones who should have been fingerprinted.

For some reason, even though I was taking care of the finances of our household all along, I felt like I needed to stay married in order to "make it." Later, I found out that other women who were in abusive marriages who are now survivors shared this same sentiment. Only when I began to look back on my journey did I realize that the financial worries, struggles, and anxieties made me feel immobile and stuck.

When you get married, you believe that your husband will provide at some level for you and your family. Even if you are financially independent, you believe that your husband will on some level contribute "his part" to the household expenses. I think this is true for most brides. If there is a time when your husband cannot contribute financially, you kick into "I'm Every Woman" mode, but you still believe that he will contribute after he "gets on his feet."

Now, I know that there are some exceptions. Sometimes, there may be physical and mental challenges. Sometimes, there may be a mutual understanding as with stay-at-home dads. If he is truly working at home taking care of the domestic affairs of the household every day, then that is a different story. For the most part, though, as long as you are married, you probably expect your husband to help you with the finances. You probably don't want to have to take care of an able-bodied man, who is your husband, for the rest of your life. Nine times out of ten, if he is not helping you with household duties at home, things probably won't end well.

On the other hand, if you are dependent on your husband financially, it does make it more challenging to leave a destructive marriage. That does not mean you have to stay. God can provide in ways that you may not have thought about. In addition, there are resources and programs available to help you gain financial independence. (See appendix B for further information.)

FEAR OF BEING ALONE

I needed to feel loved, and I craved attention from my husband. He would leave and not come home for hours and sometimes days without accounting for where he was. I spent many nights laying in the dark, wondering where he was. When he left the house, he would not tell me where he was going. Even when we went out of town together, he would leave me and go off on his own for hours.

One particular time, I wanted to just spend some time with him. He said, "I'm leaving, and I'll be back."

I asked, "Where are you going?"

He did not say anything. So, I ran outside and got in the Jeep Cherokee. He did not want me to go with him. He demanded, "Get out!" I remember how he snarled at me. I did not say anything. I just kept sitting in the passenger's seat like Rosa Parks.

In a rage, he stomped around the vehicle. He opened the door and grabbed me with all of his might. He dragged me out of the Jeep onto the concrete of the driveway. I was more embarrassed than hurt. I know the neighbors saw us scuffling. I remember looking at the back of the Jeep as it was speeding off. I got up and went back into the house and never asked where he was going ever again. I did not even want to go with him after that.

I cannot tell you why I still didn't leave. My spirit was so fragile. *I was willing to accept the crumbs of the illusion of love, and so I held out hope upon hope to truly have it one day.* There were no sweet words or nurturing body language. There were no private or public displays of affection. I only remember getting flowers from him once as a sweet gesture when we first started dating in college.

There was one other time I got flowers, when he told me that he had lost a job. I got Mother's Day cards and birthday cards from him in which he wrote, "I love you." The most disappointing birthday I had was when I did not even get a card. He verbally acknowledged it by sarcastically saying, "Oh yeah, you look good to be forty."

I don't remember him looking me in the eyes affectionately just to tell me, "I love you." There was no intimacy. I don't remember any time when I felt that he understood me or really cared about how I felt. It was always all about him and what he could get from the marriage.

If the cold loneliness I felt being married was like this, I dreaded what it must feel like being alone. I was wrong. It was as if a weight had been lifted off my shoulders when I finally decided to move on. I had been a Singles Ministry Leader in the past, and I should have identified that this was a problem that I needed to address for my own self. I don't want you to continue making this same mistake.

If you are having anxiety and worrying about "what ifs," remember that those things are not reality. They are not true. That reminds me of a common acronym for FEAR—False Evidence Appearing Real. The scripture Philippians 4:8 has since helped me to focus on positive thoughts. It says we should "think on things that are good, right, true, holy, lovely, and deserve praise. Again, think on these things."

I did not realize that my anxiety of being single again was so strong that it was keeping me immobilized. It was keeping me stuck. When I was going through that part in my journey, anxiety was a blind spot right in front of me. Even if I had a sight dog, he could not have helped me move forward.

I am not sharing this with you so that you will feel sorry for me by any means. These are moments from my journey that are in my past that I never have to experience again. I recounted them for a reason–to let you know that I understand, and that there is hope. I want you to know that if I overcame this type of mistreatment, you can, too! Jesus came to set the captive free.

YOUR DIVINE REFLECTION

The Best Lens

In your journal, write down the best lens (or scriptures) to look through in the Word of God so that you will be delivered from worry and anxiety.

Here are three examples to get you started:

1. "He has sent Me to bind up the brokenhearted, to proclaim freedom for the captives and release from darkness for the prisoners." (Isaiah 61:1b (NIV))
2. "Ask, and it will be given to you; seek, and you will find; knock and it will be opened to you. For everyone who asks receives, and the one who seeks finds, and to the one who knocks it will be opened." (Matthew 7:7-8 (NIV))
3. "Don't worry (or be anxious) about anything; instead pray about everything. Tell God what you need and thank Him for (what) He has done...And this same God who takes care of me will supply all your needs from his glorious riches, which have been given to us in Christ Jesus." (Philippians 4:6, 19 (NLT))

The Big Picture

In your journal, write your own prayer to God so that He will give you His peace and eternal view so that you will not allow anxiety to keep you from moving forward.

Here is my prayer for you:

Father God, You are all powerful and our ever-present help in the time of trouble. I lift up my sister before You today. Thank you, God, for being her provider. Thank You, Jesus, for being her Prince of Peace, and thank You, Holy Spirit, for being her Comforter. I agree with Your Word that You have not given her the spirit of fear, but of power, love, and a strong mind. I thank You for giving her Your peace that will surpass her understanding and will keep her thoughts and her heart quiet, so that she will have peaceful rest.

I agree with my sister right now that: she trusts, depends, and has her confidence in You; she chooses to think on good thoughts; and she will not choose thoughts that will cause her to worry, fret, or allow her heart to be troubled. Instead of worrying, she will pray to You about her concerns. And because her hope and expectancy are in You, Oh Lord, we thank You for the answers to her prayers in the way that You see fit. We thank You for providing all of her needs, and that she will not be in want. For this we will continue to give You our thanks and praise. In Jesus' name we pray. Amen.

Heart Vision

Close your eyes and look with your heart at what your home looks like to you now and what a quiet and peaceful, safe home looks like to you in the future. When you open your eyes, write in your journal what you saw.

Answer these questions in your journal:

1. Do you see any threats to you, or are your children in physical danger? If so, what are they? Are you being hurt emotionally? In what way?
2. How does your husband consistantly show that he wants to make changes to create a healthy relationship with you, addressing your needs and concerns?

3. What concerns do you have about other peoples' opinions of you? What about God's opinion of you?
4. In what ways do you feel loved by your husband? What are the ways that you would like to be loved?
5. Do you feel as if you are trying to fix your marriage alone? What are you doing? How would you like your husband to help? Based on how things currently are, do you really see that happening?

Shining Your Light

In this chapter, you have seen how anxiety could be a blind spot that has been limiting your mobility.

In your journal, write three things that you can do this week to let your light shine and put your heart vision into motion.

Answer these questions in your journal:

1. What can you do to have a quiet, safe, peaceful home?
2. What can you do to be true to yourself and not give others who are close to you a false impression?
3. Will you go online and order a ROUND TUIT?
4. Whom can you reach out to who will help you with your personal finances? Will you look up government agencies, associations, and "Financial Peace" classes near you?

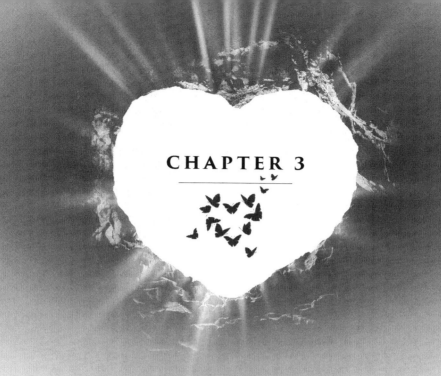

CHAPTER 3

P—Perception

PERCEPTION DECREASES PERIPHERAL VISION

Summers in Jackson, Mississippi when I was growing up were always hot and humid. The house that my dad built did not have air-conditioning. We had an attic fan, though. One extremely hot day in June of 1978, over the motor of the attic fan, I heard a knock at the front door. I was nine years old at the time, and I remember peeking out the window. I saw a skinny, black boy who was a little taller than me. We rarely had company, so I was excited to see who he was.

41

"Maybe he's a friend of Lester's," I thought. Lester is my brother who is just a year older than me. At my home, it was always just the two of us kids and my parents.

I ran and opened the door. I said, "Hi! Can I help you?"

He said, "Yes, can I come in?"

I asked, "Who are you?"

He said, "I'm Calvin, your brother."

Up until that moment, I did not know that I had any other siblings besides Lester. I was confused, but I reluctantly said, "Come on in."

He followed me into the kitchen and said to my dad, "Hi, Pops!" That was the day that I found out that my dad had been married before and I had a lot more brothers and sisters. To a nine-year-old little girl who only thought she had one brother, that was the best news ever!

Looking back on my childhood now, I realize that our family kept secrets. Not only did I not know about my family history for years, the members of our local church did not know for many more years after that. There were some things that were left unspoken. They were just not talked about. I didn't know why at the time. Now I know that it was all about *perception*. *Perception* is the third blind spot of this MAP to SEE that we will talk about in this chapter.

Many believers want other church people to see them as perfect saints. You've probably felt like that. Everyone should remember that they have missed the mark at some point and have come short of the glory of God according to Romans 3:23. Even though I grew up often hearing this scripture, I was one of those believers who acted as though I did not know it, especially when I found myself in a bad marriage.

I grew up in a time and culture where it was understood that what happened in your house stayed in your house. And it was not just my family who believed this. I have talked to other adults who have told me the same thing about their families.

Some things you just don't talk about in our society. Domestic abuse is one of those things that is kept quiet. That should not be. Silence fosters this abuse. *We need to break the silence to uncover this evil spirit that is kept hidden and allowed to lurk behind the closed doors of homes in every community. This spirit has no gender. It is neither male nor female. It is time to have an open conversation in our society about domestic abuse and how it affects everyone– both women and men.*

ABUSED MEN, SUFFERING IN SILENCE

Even though the majority of victims of domestic violence are women, there are a significant number of men who suffer in silence. According to the CDC, one in four men in the United States will be a victim of domestic violence during his lifetime. That is more than three million people every year.

I spoke to several men in confidence about their personal experience of being on the receiving end of domestic violence from their wives. The common thread and reason each of these men stated as the reason why they don't talk about how they were treated by their wives is that they do not want to be *perceived* as weak.

They told me that in our Western culture, society teaches boys that if they fall down and get scratched to get back up and brush it off and keep going. In football, they are taught that if they get hit to shake it off and keep going. Any other response in a male is seen as a sign of weakness.

One of the men that I talked to was Jeffery Harvey, who is

a behavioral health therapist at Hinds Behavioral Health Services in Jackson, MS.

He said,

> "Every person, male or female, should have the right to communicate how he or she feels without being threatened. If a man is abused by his wife, and it is talked about, what is at risk is the emasculation of the man."

He said that the majority of *physical abuse* in domestic violence occurs when the husband attacks his wife. But he also said the most common type of domestic abuse suffered by male victims was *emotional abuse* inflicted by wives on their husbands.

When the wife attacks a man's self-worth and manhood, calls him "outside of his name," isolates him from family and friends, controls and misuses the finances, and withholds affection, it makes him feel less of a person. Other men that I talked to said not only had they experienced these abuses but also the destruction of their personal property such as their computers and cell phones. Most of them said they just hide their dark secret because they considered it to be a taboo topic in society. They said that they did not know anyone to trust with this information or any place that they could turn to for help. They all agreed that they felt that the police would only belittle them for filing a report and say something like, "Man, are you for real?"

These men knew about women's shelters but didn't know of any place for men to find help. They felt that the law was biased toward women. So, several of them just internalized their pain, rejection, and bruised egos. They all distanced themselves emotionally and physically from their relationships.

Hopelessness, depression, and loneliness were the emotions that they talked about.

One of the men that I talked to said, "I am in a miserable place." He said that he thought about his children and how separation and divorce would affect them. He knew that his children saw how their mother treated him, and he worried about how that was affecting them. He said her abusive treatment of him made his children feel animosity for their mother and empathy for him. He was concerned about the behavioral patterns that both his daughters and sons were learning and how that would impact them one day when they entered adult relationships.

Harvey asked me this pointed question,

"Boys are taught not to put their 'hands on' girls, but who are teaching the girls not to put their hands on the boys? Young men are taught that their value in the relationship is from what they do and provide. They are not taught how they should expect to be treated."

Harvey went on to say,

"There is a double standard when it comes to how emotional abuse is perceived in society when it is done by a man versus when the same thing is done by a woman. If a man gets aggressive in how he talks to a woman (yells and attacks her character), that is *perceived* as emotional and verbal abuse. If a woman does the same thing to a man, it is not. It is swept under the rug with, 'Oh, she just got mad.'"

As women, we must look at ourselves in the mirror to see how we are treating our men. What are our children learning from our actions? We should encourage men to practice tempering their aggressive urges when it comes to understanding the sensitivity of women.

Some men may not be aware that how they are naturally wired to respond as a male may make women feel threatened and intimidated. If you ever get a chance to talk to a man whom you suspect may be a victim of domestic violence, understand that he would rather take that secret to the grave than to openly talk about it. If you ever get a chance to slip in a word of encouragement, let him know that it is not a sign of weakness to take care of himself. Let him know that he does not have to live life alone. There are resources for men, too. (See appendix B.) The strongest thing that he could ever do is to have enough strength to walk away from the relationship if there is no hope of repairing it when it has become destructive.

Men have feelings too, even though they may try to hide them. Everyone deserves to be loved and respected. *The social stigma of how abused men are perceived keeps them stuck in a dark place, and they may feel that they have no path forward.* They also need to look in their hearts to see what God is showing them to do.

One of these men said to me,

"I am going to get out. If another guy feels hopeless and doesn't feel like he has any options, that is not true. He has to be true to himself. I would tell him that as long as there is breath in your body, you have an option to get out. It may not be the way you want it to happen, but it may be the best way for you in the long run. It might cost you, but you always have options."

TUNNEL VISION

Not long ago, a patient came to see me for an eye exam in order to get her driver's license renewed. She gave me a form to fill out. This form has two categories to evaluate functional vision. The first one measures a person's sight looking straight ahead in each eye. The second measures a person's peripheral vision in each eye.

Looking straight ahead, the woman was able to see all of the letters on the eye chart down to the 20/20 letters in each eye. However, when I checked her peripheral vision, because of her specific eye condition, her side vision was very limited. It was as if she were looking through a toilet paper roll in each eye.

I told her, "Some people are legally blind because they cannot see half of the eye chart in their best eye. That is not the case for you. You can see directly in front of you at the eye chart just fine with both eyes. Because of the results of your peripheral vision test, however, you are legally blind."

"You mean that I have tunnel vision?" she asked.

I nodded my head yes.

She said, "I knew that I was having trouble seeing in my side vision when I was driving with my mother the other day. I almost hit a child riding his bike. He came out of nowhere right in front of me. I slammed on my breaks and barely missed him. My mom screamed, 'Didn't you see that kid??!!' "I did not see him coming from the side," she said. "I could only see right in front of me."

I told her, "It is best that you do not drive, not just for your sake, but for your mother's and for everyone else on the road."

I had to complete the form saying she was legally blind

because of her limited peripheral vision and recommend that she not drive because she did not meet public safety guidelines.

I'm mentioning this anecdote because when it comes to how we view our relationships; at times we all suffer from tunnel vision. Sometimes you don't pay any attention to those outside of your intimate relationship. Sometimes you don't even pay attention to yourself.

MY PERIPHERAL VISION

In a sense, I myself had tunnel vision. Before getting a divorce, I was only looking straight ahead at one thing—fixing my marriage. I did not consider myself. I lost sight of my own sense of self and identity. I forgot about what made me happy and what I enjoyed doing for fun. I only considered what I could do to win the approval of my husband and what would make him happy. I thought that if I could do that, maybe I would win his attention, be loved and validated.

"How did he perceive me? Why was he not looking at me affectionately? Was it because I had gained weight after having the children? How could I make him happy? What could I do to make sure I did not do anything to upset him?" were the questions that constantly bounced around in my mind.

Even though these were my thoughts, I did not look deep inside my heart. I did not acknowledge and consider my own pain and hurt. I ignored the great sacrifice I was willing to endure for the sake of being married.

Even though I was married, I felt like I was facing life alone. I did not feel my husband's love or support financially, in parenting our children, or with basic household chores. There was always something to deal with, like finding evidence of his other life outside of our marriage, of his unfaithfulness, or his flipping the discussion and falsely accusing me. In order to not feel overwhelmed, I would only deal with one thing at a time that required my immediate attention and suppressed the rest.

I did not practice healthy habits. Unfortunately, I would push back the pain and stuff it down instead of dealing with it. I would compartmentalize the hurt and disappointment. Instead of looking in my heart, I was too busy looking around outwardly, picking up the broken pieces of my life and attempting to put them back together, or I was too exhausted trying.

I knew that at any given moment, he could lose his temper. I did not like it when he yelled or confronted me in any way. I tried to keep the peace so that he would not get upset with me or the kids.

Metaphorically, what I just described to you was my tunnel vision. I didn't think about how my actions were affecting other people around me. I did not consider the toll my attempts to constantly please my husband were taking on me or how they would affect my children then, throughout their adolescent years, and in their adult lives when they have families.

As I mentioned in chapter 2, I did not tell family, friends, or people at church or work about my chaotic life at home. I was concerned about how they would perceive me if they found out. By hiding what was going on in my marriage, I distanced myself from them. I never thought my marriage was all that bad. I thought that it was something that I could handle. I always thought that it was going to get better.

Even if the people around me guessed something was not quite right, they did not question me because I was living a life of denial and not being true to myself. I would tell them and myself, "I'm fine. We are all doing good." How could anyone come into my life to help me if I kept the door to my own heart shut tight?

As I mentioned before, I believed that God was on my side, and that He was going to supernaturally work it out. I prayed that God would change my husband. My faith did not work because that was not my husband's prayer, and I had isolated myself from people. God does not intend for us to live life alone. God works through people, and He could not work through me because I did not want to make a decision to change. That meant that I did not exercise the power and authority of my free will. Until I did that, God continued to wait on me.

So, there I was, slamming on my brakes while traveling on my life's journey. *I was only looking straight ahead at my shattered marriage. I did not realize that by not focusing on myself or on the other people in my life around me and my God-given authority, I was keeping myself from moving forward.*

PERCEPTION, MORE THAN A BLIND SPOT

Perception can limit your vision by being more than a small blind spot. It can limit your entire peripheral vision. It will keep you from seeing how you are affecting others.

If you are only concerned about how your husband perceives you, you will not be concerned about your own health and well-being. You will not show yourself love and respect. Your value is not dependent on anyone's opinion of you. Your value was given to you when God created you both wonderfully and beautifully according to Psalm 139:14.

If you are only concerned about your husband's perception of you, you will not make decisions that are in the best interest of your children's development, safety, and adult behavioral patterns. You have to make a decision to break this generational hurt. Even after getting a divorce, my children had to go through counseling and treatment for depression and anger management that were directly associated with my unhealthy relationship with their father.

If you are always portraying a false perception that everything is all right to others in your life, you could be cutting off those who could be your support system. If you are not truthful to people in your immediate family, close friends, or a trusted godly brother or sister at church, you could be limiting the hand that God can work through to help you on your path forward. There are no perfect saints. Remember that no church is perfect because imperfect people make up the church congregation.

You don't have to pretend any longer. God sees you. He knows what you are going through, and He is waiting on you to be true to your heart and choose life for yourself and your children. If you or your children are being abused verbally, mentally, emotionally, financially, sexually, or physically in your own home, you should never keep silent and stay in that unsafe environment.

After I decided to get a divorce, I did not let the feelings of fear and embarrassment keep me from getting help anymore. I confided in my parents, pastor's wife, and three close friends. They listened to me, prayed with me, and counseled me. They helped me to deal with the pain that I had been carrying around for years. They encouraged me to move on and were a very important support system as I made a transition to a new life.

At this time more than any, be open to allow the people that God puts in your life to help you. Pray that God will bring people across your path at the right time. Look for those people who genuinely care about you, will not be judgmental, will actively listen to you, and be there for you when you need them. Look for people who are not controlling but allow you to make your own decisions about what will be best for you and your children.

If you are concerned about how people will perceive you for making a decision to change your life for the better, ask yourself, "What does it matter what they think anyway?" They don't know what you went through. They are not living your life, and their opinions will not change a thing. People will always have opinions no matter what you do. At the end of the day, if you are true to yourself and God, that is all that matters. The Word of God says in 3 John 1:2 that "He wishes above all things that you prosper, and be in health, even as your soul (mind, emotions, and will) prospers." The only approval that matters is God's approval.

YOUR DIVINE REFLECTION

The Best Lens

In your journal, write down the best lens (or scriptures) to look through in the Word of God so that you will not be limited by the tunnel vision that can come from your perception and the perception of others.

Here are three examples to get you started:

1. "Work hard so you can present yourself to God and receive His approval." 2 Timothy 2:15a (NLT)
2. "Your beauty will make the king desire you." Psalm 45:11a (GNT)
3. "Does this sound as if I am trying to win human approval? No indeed! What I want is God's approval! Am I trying to be popular with people? If I were still trying to do so, I would not be a servant of Christ." Galatians 1:10 (GNTD)

The Big Picture

In your journal, write your own prayer to God so that you will receive the perception that He has of you. Ask Him for His eternal view so that you will not have any problem seeing the people in your peripheral vision.

Here is my prayer for you:

Father God, You alone are holy, and You know everything about my sister. You desire that she is truthful and honest in the inward parts of her heart. Help her to be honest with herself so that she can identify what is going on in her life and what she wants for herself and her family.

Help her to make wise decisions for her life. Help her to know how precious she is in your sight, how much You love her with Your everlasting love, and that You will see that her needs are met. Let her be open to the people that You will send across her path that will give her Your wise counsel, lift her up, and help her. All these things I ask in Jesus' name. Amen

Heart Vision

Take a deep breath. This exercise will not be easy, but you can do it if you really want things to change. Close your eyes and look with your heart to see how your perception of yourself and others' perceptions of you are contributing to where you are today on your life's journey. What painful things have you decided to endure at your own expense for the sake of your marriage? What things are you embarrassed about and don't want people to know that are going on in your life or home? When you open your eyes, write in your journal what you saw. Answer these questions in your journal:

1. Describe yourself. Do you perceive yourself as valuable, or do you doubt your own value? Why or Why not?
2. What don't you like about how your husband treats you and your children?
3. How do you feel about how your husband treats you and your children?
4. How do you think others perceive you and your family?
5. How do you feel about other people's perceptions of you and your family?
6. How does trying to pretend everything is okay make you feel; stressful?

7. What other person besides the one you mentioned in chapter 1 can you trust, who won't judge you, and whom you feel you can pray with and talk to about your marriage?

Shining Your Light

Hopefully, in this chapter you have learned how your perception or other people's perceptions can be a blind spot that can limit your ability to move forward. By identifying this potential obstacle, you can then consider what you can do about it.

In your journal, write three things that you can do this week to let your light shine and to put your heart vision into motion.

Answer these questions in your journal:

1. When can you make an appointment to talk to the person you named during your heart vision exercise? Talk to this individual in confidence (whatever you are comfortable sharing) about what is going on with you in your marriage. Tell this individual that you are not looking for advice but just someone to listen and support you. Ask this individual to pray with you, that you make the best decision concerning your marriage.
2. Do something special for yourself because you deserve it. What will it be?
3. Look for a man (among your family, friends, and coworkers) who may need you to encourage him to seek help if he is in a toxic relationship. Will you pray for discernment and be more sensitive to who this man (and other men) may be?
4. Set aside fifteen minutes to look at *Grace for Purpose's* YouTube Video that was published on April 1, 2019. In

this video, Lisa Bevere talks about perceptions—God's, yours, and others. It's called "You Are Worth More Than You Think, Woman of God." When can you look at it?

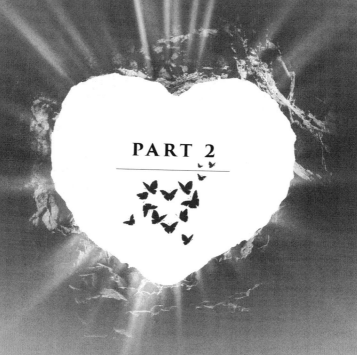

PART 2

S.E.E.

CHAPTER 4

S—Spirit

SPIRIT VISION SHOWS YOU WHAT YOUR EYES WON'T

It was in the fall of 2006. It was one of those Sunday mornings that I found myself rushing to get to church on time with my two children. My son was nine years old, and my daughter was eleven at the time. We were running extremely late, but I was determined to at least get there to hear the sermon.

We finally made it to the sanctuary of Rhema Bible Church in Broken Arrow, Oklahoma. There were no end seats available, so we had to slide in front of a few people to find three seats in the balcony. Pastor Kenneth Hagin Jr. was already preaching. He said, "You are a spirit. You have a soul. And you live in a body." That struck a huge chord with me. His message came from I Thessalonians 5:23:

> "May the God who gives us peace make you holy in every way and keep your whole being – spirit, soul, and body – free from every fault at the coming of our Lord Jesus Christ."

I sat there and listened to the rest of his sermon. He said,

> "Your body has senses that help you to make contact with the outside world around you. Your soul is the part of you that is your mind, emotions, and your will. Your spirit is the real you on the inside. Your life and breath. It is the part of you that makes contact with God and where He makes contact with you."

Church dismissed, and my children and I went back home. But I never forgot what the pastor said in that sermon.

When I was nine years old, I asked Jesus to come into my heart (my spirit) and become the Lord and Savior of my life. The Holy Spirit came to live in my spirit, or you may say in my heart. It is from this place in my heart that my spirit (my inner person) prays to God. This is important because until I heard that sermon, the only perspective of how my life looked in the outside world around me (especially at home) was from my physical eyes. They served as the part of my body's senses that were only showing me one dimension—the physical dimension. Others around me could see my life better than I could see it myself. But I was trying hard not to show any signs of the dysfunction in my home.

My spirit was praying to God from my perspective of what I could see with my physical eyes and how I mentally visualized having a better marriage, but I was not allowing my spirit to catch God's vision and perspective of what my life looked like to Him. I was not seeing in the spiritual dimension. My physical eyes could not show me the invisible, spiritual things that were missing in my life. Only the eyes of my spirit—or the eyes of my heart—could do that.

Keeping the eyes of your spirit closed is the fourth blind spot of this MAP to SEE that we talk about in this chapter. We will talk about opening the eyes of your heart to see with your spirit. This is spirit vision. This is heart vision.

FORGOTTEN DREAMS

When I was a little girl growing up in Jackson, Mississippi I would close my eyes and see myself standing before others and teaching them. I played with a lot of dolls. On sunny days, I would put them all in a toy baby stroller and go outside under a shade tree in the yard. I would take them out and line them up in a row and pretend to teach them their lessons for the day.

Some days, I pretended to be their mom. Other days, I pretended to be their grade schoolteacher or even their Sunday schoolteacher. I had some white chalk, a small chalkboard, and a small towel for an eraser. The lesson for the day was either ABCs, 123s, or Genesis.

You see, my dad was a public speaker. He would begin one particular speech with, "In the beginning, God...." Now looking back on that time in my life, I see that God was showing me an image in my spiritual vision of what I would be doing later in my life. I became my children's first teacher as my mom did and as you may have to. I became a children's, preteen, and youth Sunday schoolteacher. I became a lay speaker and now, a motivational speaker.

When I was an adult and a student at the University of Alabama School of Optometry, I would close my eyes and visualize what my own optometry practice would look like. On a piece of paper, I drew out the plans that I saw in my spirit. I shared the floor plans that I drew up with my dad. The plans included a waiting area, front desk, optical exam lanes, imaging room, lab, break room, and even bathrooms. I worked as an optometrist for other doctors in over twenty different locations, among three different states, for nearly twenty years before that dream of having my own practice with a very similar floor plan that I had dreamed of manifested itself. That is where I am working today.

You have the amazing ability to close your physical eyes and see what's inside your heart. Through faith, you can see things that God has in store for you before they become a reality. God can give you dreams, and He can show you images of things to come.

During the dark years of my abusive marriage, I no longer saw those images. I no longer dreamed dreams of a bright future. I only existed alone in silence and shame. If this is you, and you find yourself here at this point of your MAP to SEE, close your physical eyes and open the eyes of your heart, and ask God to help you to see what He sees for your life. Think back to the time before your destructive marriage. Revisit your dreams.

INVISIBLE FRUIT

As I said in chapter 1, when your life is honoring Christ, you will bear spiritual fruit. When the Holy Spirit comes into your heart, He gives you character traits called the fruit of the Spirit. These character traits have to grow and develop and be nurtured and cultivated in the right environment for them to mature and be enjoyed. You have to cut off what is hindering you from bearing God's invisible fruit. According to Matthew 7:18-20,

> "A good tree cannot bear bad fruit, and a bad tree cannot bear good fruit. Every tree that does not bear good fruit is cut down and thrown into the fire. Thus, by their fruit you will recognize them."

If you ask Him, God will show you in your spiritual vision the spiritual fruit that He wants to manifest in your life so that you can enjoy it. I mention "spiritual fruit" again in this chapter because they are invisible to your physical eyes. *Your natural eyes cannot see love, peace, and joy. You can see and feel the byproducts of them, however. These invisible things are the things that will bring you well-being and true happiness.*

You may have to prune and separate yourself from what is not allowing this fruit to grow. In order to do this, I got a divorce. You may have to separate yourself from an abuser so that you can see things more clearly. You may have to seek protection. If you do, make sure you have a safe plan. (See appendix B for a resource on safe planning.) You have to be in an environment that allows God's light to give you unhindered nourishment for spiritual fruit to grow.

You may have to be "repotted." You may have to move from a threatening environment. It is best to surround yourself with people who will help cultivate these spiritual character traits. This is what I did when I moved back to my home state of Mississippi after getting a divorce. Because I had been isolated from them, I had to work on growing relationships with my support system—close family, friends, and other believers.

A lot of people think they have success when they actually see the physical fruits of their labor in worldly prosperity like a new house or a new car or a new job or money. There is nothing wrong with these things in and of themselves. But they alone are not abundant life.

I had those things before when I was in my destructive marriage, but I did not experience life more abundantly. Now that I am enjoying the unseen spiritual fruit that can only be seen with my spiritual eyes, I can "taste and see that the Lord is good." When you can experience the fruit of the Spirit, you are experiencing your promise of having an abundant life (John 10:10). This is God's vision for your life. Where you find this fruit, you will find your promised land, and you can enter into your peaceful, restful place.

When you are in an abusive marriage, your life is anything but peaceful. Oh, you may have times were there is quiet before the storm, but you never know when the hurricane is going to blow through. When you are in denial, you rationalize your abuser's behavior by saying, "He is really a good person. He is not always like that." The problem with that statement is *he should never be like that.* You may rationalize why you stay because you may love the part of him that can be kind and charismatic. Everyone has their own reasons. Let me give you some insight into mine.

THE FIRST REASON WHY I STAYED

After getting a restraining order and filing for divorce, my mom asked me the common question that many survivors of domestic violence are asked, "Why did you stay so long?" She asked me this after I had finally broken through the denial and the silence and moved back to Jackson, Mississippi. I did not know that abuse flourishes in silence. She said, "If I was being abused, I would have left."

Well, it's not that easy.

The answer was—*first of all*—I did not see myself as an abused woman. I was blind to reality. Lord knows, I had plenty of other reasons to leave my husband, but the word "abuse" never crossed my mind as a reason. I did not know the warning signs or patterns of an abuser. I did not stop and realize that the man whom I thought was my soul mate, the father of my children, was abusing me.

I was too busy looking at my circumstances with my natural eyes and trying to fix everything. I was busy trying to keep the family together. I was busy trying to run with the vision that I had for my life. I was too busy trying to pretend to others that everything was okay.

I was even busier trying to do what I thought a woman of God was supposed to do: staying committed to her vows—for better or WORSE, being the praying wife, giving up what I wanted, and trying to be in agreement with what I could to please God. And while it is right to try to do all of those things, I did not realize that those principles don't apply to an abusive marriage, and I did not realize that I had one. I did not know what an abusive relationship looked like.

Now hindsight is 20/20. After getting a divorce and learning about abusive relationships, I see that during the twenty years of my relationship with my husband, I lived in a typical, continuous cycle of abuse.

I didn't realize how *others* saw me until that dark night that

I told you about in chapter 2 when the police officer gave me that card with a crisis hotline number and details on how to contact a women's shelter. At the time, I did not take time to process the gravity of it all. I just knew I had to get out of there with my children.

Until that night, my physical eyes just wouldn't show me what my life really looked like. I had to open the eyes of my heart to see what was happening to me and my children on the inside. As I've said already, when I closed the door and turned around and saw the fear in my children's eyes, that was the day I made the decision that I had to make a change.

That dark night before the break of day, in my spirit, I saw where I was, and I saw what I had to do to get out with my children. Until then, *I had been living with a blind spot in my spirit's ability to see myself clearly. There was a space in my spiritual heart that had been hurting for so long that I did not acknowledge its presence.* I had been subconsciously suppressing my emotional pain so much that it had become "normal." Everything else in my life surrounded and camouflaged it. But that night, it had been revealed. Seeing it was one thing. Accepting it was another.

You do not believe a thing if you don't even know that it exists or understand it. When you do find out about it and understand it, you can then believe it. Through faith, in your spirit you can then see in the spiritual realm what you want to manifest in the physical realm.

Before you can change anything and move forward in your life, you have to first see where you are now. Only then can you see where you need to go.

THE SECOND REASON WHY I STAYED

The second reason why it was difficult for me to leave my marriage was because I felt that it would be dangerous! Before the police officers left, and I saw that they were going to take my husband to jail, I said to one of the officers, "Oh no, I am in trouble now."

He said, "Why do you say that? This is not your fault."

I said, "You don't understand, *everything is always my fault* according to him."

He said, "As a husband and father, I am sad to see that you are afraid of the man who is supposed to be nurturing and protecting you...the man that you call your husband."

I was most terrified after I had left my husband and he had gotten out of jail. He pulled some wires out from under the hood of the vehicle that I was driving so that it would not run. When I went to service the vehicle, I was shocked to find out my name was not on the title because my funds had been used to purchase it. I found myself without transportation. I was too afraid to go back to our home. In effect, I had become homeless.

After my husband continued to stalk me, I asked people who I worked with to let me stay with them. I found the courage to finally reach out for help. I was in the state of Oklahoma, far away from lifelong friends and family, but I had people around me who cared. *I needed this reality check to make me look into my heart of hearts.* Other people around me looked into their hearts, too and had compassion for me.

First, my employer let me stay with him. His neighbor said that he had seen my husband's car slowly coming down the street several times. I knew that he was looking for me, and that I could not stay there. I continued to look over my shoulder, stay in different places, ride in different vehicles, and walk to where I needed to go, pulling my suitcase behind me.

This reminds me of one particular time when I had just finished doing Lasek Refractive Surgery on two of my patients. I walked out of the operating room of Tulsa Laser Center. I grabbed my suitcase and overnight bag and started pulling them behind me as I left the building and started walking down the street. I walked ten blocks to where I knew a church member lived. I was glad when she answered the door. I was even happier when she took me in for the night.

I stayed with three different coworkers, my good friend and hair stylist, and a friend of my employer took me into her home without even knowing me. It was so humbling, and I was so grateful because although I was a stranger, she took me in. As the weeks passed, I could not continue to evade my husband this way. I decided to rejoin my children in my home state of Mississippi a few weeks earlier than I had planned.

I returned to my parents' home where I had taken my children the previous month for their safety. When I got there, they were still afraid. They did not even want to go outside. My daughter repeatedly wanted to sleep with me because she was having nightmares. She had to have treatment for anxiety and depression some years later. My son was just angry.

My son developed aggressive tendencies because, as he later told me, "I never wanted to feel like I did the night that we left our home in Oklahoma, and I never wanted to be bullied again by anyone." I reassured my children, but I did not let on that I, too was still on edge and in fear because I kept seeing in my mind's eye the contempt on my husband's face when he told me a few weeks earlier, "I am going to take care of you!" I also thought about how he had put a gun to my head six years earlier. I could not take any more chances. I knew that I had to continue working my safety plan.

So, I got a gun permit. Even though I had a restraining order, I started keeping a weapon with me for protection. Today, I know the facts about abused women, and that I am one of the blessed ones who can call herself a survivor. I now realize that the most dangerous time for me was after I had ended my relationship. It is during this time that many abused women are killed. Let us always honor and remember their memory.

THE THIRD REASON WHY I STAYED

And finally, it was difficult to leave because I was strapped for cash. The financial abuse had drained me of all of my reserves. I alone had paid the bills and other family expenses before, during, and after my divorce. With the divorce, there were travel costs, relocation and moving expenses, attorney and other legal fees. This was not the first time I had lost my house, my car, and my job because of the relationship. But this time, I felt like I was at ground zero. That was the lowest time in my life, and I was in my dark place.

I filed for divorce, but I was not getting any child support. In fact, I did not get any child support until three years after the divorce when I got a garnishment order, which, of course, involved paying more legal fees. I had to wait three more years for arrears payments to begin because my now ex-husband falsely denied that he owed them.

I remembered the sermon that Pastor Hagin had preached, "I am a spirit. I have a soul. And I live in a body." My body was tired and weak. My mind and my emotions of my soul were weary, but my will and spirit still had hope in God. With my spirit vision, I could see the light at the end of the tunnel.

FOCUSING SPIRITUAL VISION

As a professional optometrist, I use lenses every day to bend light to focus it on a place in the back of the eye called the *retina*. This process is called *refraction*. In the best-case scenario, when light is focused on a particular place on the retina, called the *macula*, you see clearly.

If you look through the lens of the Word of God, it will bend the light of God through the eyes of your spirit so that you will be able to see the things of God more clearly.

Just as you can decide what you are going to continue to look at and focus on with your physical eyes, you can decide what you are going to continue to look at and focus on with your spiritual eyes. Just as there are resources to help you navigate everyday life, there are resources to help you navigate your spiritual life if you focus on them.

You may have been blind to your reality like I was, and now you may see that you need to make a change. The most important resource that can help your spiritual eyes to see who you are, what God wants for you, and how to go about taking your next step is the Word of God. I had been reading the Word of God my whole life, but my spiritual growth was stuck in this area because of my lack of understanding.

With my blind spots no longer blocking my spiritual view, my bible study and prayers reached a new level. The same scriptures that I knew on peace, anxiety, God's love for me, His provision, and wisdom took on a whole new meaning. I continued to meditate on these scriptures. I read, memorized, and confessed them to continue to build my faith. I began to see myself receiving what the scriptures said I should be receiving before they actually happened. My spiritual eyes began to see clearer as I looked through the perfect lens of the Word of God. I began to see myself better from God's point of view.

As a believer, you can ask the Holy Spirit to lead you to the perfect scripture appropriate for the situation you are going through. You can ask the Holy Spirit to teach you so that you can understand the wonderful treasures that are hidden in the Word of God for you to discover. If you do this and apply what you discover to your life, you will be able to enjoy the invisible fruit of the Spirit yourself and not just be a giver of it. Go ahead and start dreaming the dreams again that God put in your spirit years ago before your toxic relationship.

As you look into your own heart and take a self-assessment, seek God's perspective of your life, then your spirit vision can help you see clearer why you don't have to stay entangled in the web of an abusive marriage. You alone have to make that choice with your own God-given, free will. After finally making *your own* decision, you can more confidently take action and step out in faith.

YOUR DIVINE REFLECTION

The Best Lens

In your journal, write down the best lens (or scriptures) to look through in the Word of God so that you will not only depend on your physical eyes to see what things really look like. Use this spiritual perspective to ground yourself as you look at the circumstances of your marriage with your spirit vision.

Here are three examples to get you started:

1. "Open the eyes of their hearts *and let the light of Your truth flood in*. Shine Your light on the hope You are calling them to embrace. Reveal to them the glorious riches You are preparing as their inheritance." Ephesians 1:18 (Voice)
2. "Indeed, our lives are guided by faith (eyes of faith, spiritual vision), not by sight (physical eyesight)." 2 Corinthians 5:7 (GW)
3. "So, we do not focus on what is seen, but on what is unseen. For what is seen is temporary, but what is unseen is eternal." 2 Corinthians 4:18 (HCSB)

The Big Picture

In your journal, write your own prayer to God that He will give you His eternal view of your marriage and clarify your spiritual vision concerning what you should do about it.

Here is my prayer for you:

Father God, You are sovereign. You are spirit. And we recognize who You are, and we honor You with our whole hearts. God, You see and search our hearts. Whatever You find that is not clean, we ask that You take it away and give us a clean heart. Renew a right spirit within us. From her clean heart, and her renewed spirit is the place where my sister connects with You, God.

Through faith, open the eyes of her heart so that she will see herself as You see her. Help her to see her life from Your perspective. Remind her of the wonderful dreams that You put in her heart years ago that You still want to manifest in her life. Show her the true fruit that her husband is or is not bearing from his spirit. Show her the spiritual fruit that You want her to enjoy.

Reveal any blind spots that she may have in her heart that she cannot see about herself. If she is being abused, let her see it for what it is. If she feels as if her life is in danger, protect her and help her to find a support person who will help her to establish a safe plan of escape. If she needs money to move forward with her plan to leave, show her what she needs to do so that You can help provide the financial assistance that is available to her.

Show her in Your Word and in her spirit the next steps that she should take daily concerning her marriage and family. All these things I ask in Jesus' name. Amen.

Heart Vision

Close your eyes and look in your heart so that you can see how healthy your spirit is on the inside. Does it look strong, cheerful, and growing, or does it look weak, sad, and crushed? When you open your eyes, write a detailed description of what you saw in your journal, and why.

Answer these questions in your journal:

1. Are you certain that your heart is connected to God so that you can communicate with each other freely?
2. Are you being led by your spirit, or are you allowing your soul (your thoughts and emotions) and how you feel in your body to lead you?
3. What dreams that you had in your heart for yourself have you stopped dreaming about?
4. What are the biggest challenges you have that would prevent you from deciding to get out of a relationship that is hurting you and your children?

Shining Your Light

In this chapter, you have seen how being sensitive to your spirit can reveal things that your natural eyes will not show you. Some of these things can be blind spots that keep you from moving on in your life beyond abuse and into your purpose and can only be revealed by your spiritual vision.

In your journal, write three things that you can do this week to let your light shine and put your heart vision into motion. Answer these questions in your journal:

1. What can you do each day to make sure your spirit is in fellowship with God? (See appendix C if you need help with this answer.)
2. What can you do or to whom can you talk to help put you on the right track to making at least one of your dreams come true?
3. What will you do to face one of the challenges that is causing you to stay where you are?

E—Enabling

ENABLING WON'T GIVE YOU THE RESPECT YOU DESERVE

There was once a man who was always running late for work. Every morning, he would speed pass a policewoman who was always parked in the same place right after the speed limit sign. Two weeks went by, and the policewoman did not stop him for speeding. Each morning for the next two weeks she would turn on her blue warning lights as he sped by her, but that is all she did.

He always looked back in his rearview mirror after he passed her, but she never pursued him, so he kept speeding by her without consequence. One morning after he zoomed by, she not only turned on her blue lights, she turned on her siren and sped after him. He was shocked. He got angry and pulled over.

When she walked up to the side of his car, she said, "Let me see your driver's license and proof of insurance."

He handed them over to her and asked, "What did I do wrong?"

She said, "You were speeding."

He blurted out, "You did not stop me one time during the last month when I have been speeding by. Why did you stop me this time?"

She shouted back, "Oh, so you knew you were speeding all last month! At first, I just gave you the benefit of the doubt. But then it became a habit. So, why didn't you ever slow down and respect the law? Even though I did not stop you, did that make it right?"

"No," he replied, "that did not make it right...but I did not slow down because you let me keep going every time. That is why I did not respect you."

She finished writing his speeding ticket and snapped back, "You may not respect me, but it will be in your best interest to respect this."

She handed him the ticket. She got back in her police car and drove off. This policewoman was an enabler. She allowed this man to continue to break the law without consequence. Since she was a police officer, she had the authority to stop him every time he was speeding, but she didn't. This violation went on until she decided to demand respect.

In this chapter, we discuss how you can be blind to the fact that not demanding respect enables your abuser. We will now talk about the blind spot of enabling on your MAP to SEE your path forward.

THE LAST SUPPER

In April of 2001, I asked my first accountant to meet me for dinner at a nice restaurant in Montgomery, Alabama one day after work. He agreed without hesitation. We ordered our food from the menu and started eating.

He asked, "Why did you ask me out to dinner?"

I said, "I want to discuss the monthly fees that you have been charging my account for several years. I noticed that the only activity on my statements are in the month of April when you prepare my yearly taxes. What do you have to say about that?"

He answered, "I kept billing you because you let me."

"Well," I said, "consider this month's bill for this year's taxes paid in full due to the credit you owe me from my overpayment over the years."

"You got me," he said as he finished eating. "Is this my last supper?" he asked with a sarcastic grin.

With a face like stone, I said, "Yes, it is." I paid the check and left.

This was one example of how I enabled (or allowed) someone to take advantage of me financially. Let me give you another example.

DOG FOOD

During the same period this accountant was cheating me out of my money, my employer was paying me as a contract laborer. This meant that I paid my own taxes. I did not have any expenses to write off, so I only made two-thirds of what I was paid. I did not get a raise during the nearly ten-year period I worked there. I got paid as if I were a salaried employee. It did not matter how many hours I worked during or outside of office hours. And unfortunately for me, I did not ask to be compensated for all the extra work that I was doing.

After my employer started holding my check because of other expenses that he had to pay, I put in my thirty-day notice.

He asked me, "Why are you quitting?"

I said, "Because you are not paying me fairly."

He told me, "Well, you let me. I fed you dog food before, and you ate it."

I felt no emotion when he said this. I simply walked out of his office.

I share these stories with you because I want you to see the three words that each of these stories have in common: "You let me." Not only was I disrespected in the workplace, I was also disrespected at home. Now, looking back on my life's journey, I can see how my ex-husband could have used these same three words as well.

Even though it was not my fault that my ex-husband abused me, I do realize that I did have a part to play in my relationship during those twenty years of marriage. I mentioned in chapter 4 some of the reasons *why* I stayed regardless of the fact that I was in a dark, painful place. But I had to ask myself, "*What* did I do all of those years that kept me in the marriage?" My role was the enabler.

Just like the policewoman in the opening story, I made excuses. I got defensive when confronted. I did not prioritize myself or my needs. I failed to provide or follow through with consequences for the bad behavior of others. As with my accountant and past employer, I was not able to display emotion, and

I did not set boundaries for myself. Because I did all of these things in my marriage, I did not demand respect. I allowed my ex-husband to continue his abusive behavior for years.

NOT ACKNOWLEDGING

I did not acknowledge to myself that my husband was mistreating me. I did not miss any public displays of affection because there were no private ones. I ignored the negative comments he made about me. I brushed it off by saying he was just having a bad day. I turned a blind eye to his absence in our home. I told myself, I was the home body.

I continued to make excuses for his not taking responsibility. There were many excuses I made throughout the journey of my abusive relationship. See if you can find them:

I justified my relationship by thinking about how it started out when he was kind, charming, and funny. We shared the same Christian family background; we were college alumni from Ole Miss, and we had the same future goals. He treated me as if I were a queen. Sounds like the perfect guy, right?

So, we got married, and I thought we would live happily ever after. We moved out of Mississippi two different times in our marriage for school and work, isolating me from friends and family....**But** at the time I never thought about that. His infidelity broke trust....**But** I wanted to fight for my marriage.

He threatened my life....**But** I was a strong woman who was living with a troubled man, and I was the one he depended on and the one who could help him. At one point, he said he felt like committing suicide, and he was just not thinking straight.... **But** I could not leave him because I was the one who encouraged him since he had refused to get professional counseling.

Earlier in our marriage, he had taken our children from me to live in another state to get me to give him money and to force me to go there to live with him....**But** he brought them back to me when his plan did not work. He would easily get angry and out of control. He would yell and smash and break things.... **But** I was the quiet, calm one who was able to deal with it, clean it up, and make things right each time. He was the one who repeatedly brought up "divorce" .... **But** I was the one who kept asking, "Why did you say that? I don't want a divorce."

We had a lot of storms in our marriage....**But** he would always say how sorry he was and that he would not do it again. I don't know how many times he lied and told me, "I'm going to give you the money back," when I found out that he had taken my money, or maxed out a credit card in my name that I did not know about, or demanded that I or our children give him more money even though he was not accountable or responsible with the finances.

He would come up with crazy, elaborate stories that kept my mind spinning....**But** I was the one who had to be level-headed and be there to fix it. No matter what the circumstances were, if I ever asked him to be accountable, he would not give an account. He would turn the tables on me, and say, "You are always trying to start something" .... **But** I second-guessed and told myself, "Maybe he is right."

He was always dressed to the nines, and his shirts were heavily starched from the cleaners....**But** I did not make any special effort to look cute because I did not have any shopping money left, and besides, I did not feel special after all of the sarcastic put-downs that he made about my appearance. And then there were his repeated false accusations that I was cheating on him.

NOT ME!

In chapter 2, I told you about that dark night of the last day that my husband and I were together. It was after midnight when he hit me and pinned our daughter to the floor as my son stood there frozen in fear. It was not until after calling the police that reality set in. That's when the police officer gave me a card to go to a shelter for battered women.

I balked at the notion and was almost offended that he had even given me that card. I exclaimed, "I am **not** a battered woman!"

He just stood there and looked at me, and said, "I see this all the time."

So, I was in denial. I did not have time to process everything at the time. I just knew that I had to get out of my home with my children. We fled our home to get to safety. The next day, I filed for divorce.

During the course of the next week, I found myself sitting in a different office down the hall talking to a new attorney, not the one I had previously spoken to and related the history of my marriage.

My new attorney said, "Because of the nature of your circumstances, my partner reassigned your case to me because I specialize in representing battered women."

Again, I got defensive. I leaned forward toward her and insisted, "I am **not** a battered woman! Yes, my husband hit me... **but** that was the first time that happened. I was afraid to stay at the house because I did not know what he would do to us when he came back home. He was out of control. He was just not thinking straight."

As I listened to the words coming out of my mouth, I sat back in my seat.

She said, "I looked over your file, and what you have reported shows all of the signs of battered woman's syndrome."

I objected, "I don't have any bruises or broken limbs. I don't appreciate you judging me and my husband. I just need to do this to protect myself and my children."

There was a long pause, then it was as if she looked through me into my eyes from across her desk, and she said, **"Your husband does not love you."**

I argued back, "You do not know my husband."

She said, "Love does not hurt. If he loved you, he would not continue to hurt you without regard."

Then she pulled out a checklist of signs of emotional abuse (see appendix A). She went on to ask me a long list of questions, and to my surprise, I answered yes to nearly every one of them.

When she finished, she said, "There is such a thing as emotional abuse. What you have just reported is that YOUR EMOTIONAL SELF is so beaten up and abused that if I could see that part of you, you would not be recognizable."

I was not aware of what emotional abuse looked like. I found out that my marriage was a textbook image of it. I saw myself in each spoke in the cycle of abuse. The very fact that I was immediately getting angry and defensive was a dead giveaway that I was feeling uncomfortable with the notion that I may have been enabling my husband's abusive behavior.

NOT SETTING BOUNDARIES OR CONSEQUENCES

When we first got married, we did not go through premarital counseling. We did not talk about our likes and dislikes, come to agreements about our expectations, what we would not tolerate or what we would do if those agreements were broken. This is called setting boundaries and consequences. This step is very important in healthy relationships.

I simply expected my husband to treat me how I treated him, with respect and regard to his feelings. When that did not happen, I was disappointed because my expectations were not met. I then ended up *reacting* to what was happening to me. On the other hand, when you set boundaries for yourself, you are being *proactive*.

Setting boundaries for myself in my marriage would have involved having the following conversations:

I should have said,

- "I would like for you to be considerate of my feelings, including letting me know where you are so that I won't be worrying about you."
- "I don't feel secure when you continue to withdraw large sums out of our joint banking account. That's the account I need to pay our bills, and you're not contributing to it."
- "When you yell, turn over things, and smash things in the house, I don't feel safe. I don't feel like we have a safe zone to talk freely about our problems."

Setting consequences for my husband would have looked like this:

I should have said,

- "If you refuse to be accountable about your time outside of our home, I will not continue to live with you."
- "If you continue to spend the money that I alone am

contributing to the joint account and overdrawing it, I will close that account and open one in my own name."

- "If you can't talk about our problems calmly, I will leave you."

Since I hadn't done this early on in my marriage, I allowed the abuse to continue. I did not want to face the reality of the possibility of more pain and hurt for myself. As I explained in chapter 2, when we first got married, my husband had a job and took care of us financially. Then there were many years when he did not work. When he did start working again, he did not significantly help me financially.

At first, I was trying to help him, but then it turned into my enabling his irresponsible behavior. The Word of God says that if you don't work, you should not eat. It also says that you should bear your own burden, and if you don't provide for your own home, you are worse off than a person who does not believe in God. *So clearly, not taking care of your responsibility is a sin. So habitually aiding in such behavior is being an accomplice.*

Understand there is a difference between unconditional love and enabling. *Unconditional love* is when you decide to love without expecting anything in return for your love. You help people when they cannot do things for themselves. You cross the line to *enabling* when you are doing things for people who are able to do them for themselves.

Enabling is action in the name of love that ends up with your compensating for someone else. You either ignore his or her immature actions or you ignore the fact that the person isn't meeting his or her responsibilities, and then you take on what the person is supposed to be doing.

Not Following Through with Consequences

Now later on, I did respond with consequences, as the police-woman did in the story at the opening of this chapter. I eventually changed the locks of our home, closed our joint bank account, and left the marriage. My husband had refused to go to professional counseling a few months before I left. He told me that he did not need to go.

Before I changed the locks of our home, *my husband continued* to come in and out at all times of the day and night without regard to how I felt, *even with my asking him not to.* I finally set this boundary; *but I did not follow through with a consequence because I did not want to deal with his strife and retaliation.* He had no regard to my requests. He did not respect my feelings. When I asked him to be accountable, he would push back, start an argument, flip the blame on me and say, "You are always starting something! You don't need to know that. I am tired of you accusing me."

Even after I closed the joint checking account, he would still come home and demand money from me. *By my continuing to give in and give him money, because I didn't want him to get more upset with me, he continued to control me.* Instead of letting God work in this situation, I intervened so that my husband did not suffer the consequences of his actions and so that I would not get the backlash. This was not what I should have done. I should have stepped back, got out of the way, and let God work. If a person is comfortable, he is not motivated to change his behavior.

Although I had asked my husband to go to professional counseling for his destructive behavior, he did not go. He did not want to receive anyone's advice. *Because I did not leave then, he continued to make me and my children afraid of him until the day we left.* After he got served with the divorce papers and the restraining order, he did not want to adhere to any type of discipline. So, he continued to make threatening phone calls and stalk me, terrorizing me.

He did this because he must have believed that his tactics would work. It was not until I fled the state that I was free. Even with miles between us, at first, I was still paranoid that he would show up at any time. I kept a copy of my restraining order with me, practiced shooting my gun at the firing range, and tried to keep a low profile.

I felt quite awkward when my pastor saw me at the DMV getting my gun permit. He knew I was not getting it for hunting deer. He simply said, "Daughter, make an appointment to come see me." When I did see him in his office, he told me to start confessing Psalm 91 every day. When I did, I felt the peace of God rest in my heart. But I still carried my gun.

When you get to the point that you make the decision that you are DONE, you have to be ready with a plan or strategy to deal with the negative consequences that you may experience from your decision. But know that it is always worth it to love yourself enough to demand respect. If you don't take care of you, then who will?

Not Making Yourself a Priority

"You are never happy. No matter where you go, or what you do, you always find fault in it. What would make you happy? Is there a dream that you have that has not been fulfilled? Is there somewhere that you want to go? Is there something that you want to do?" is what I asked my husband in the fall of 2004.

He told me that he wanted to change careers and go to a school in Oklahoma. I made what he wanted my priority. Isn't that what a good wife is supposed to do? I looked for a job in Oklahoma. I got one. I resigned from the job where I was working in Mississippi and packed up everything we had. However, we had to put our plans on hold after my husband spent the relocation money.

Two years later, I tried it again. This time we made it. But when we got there, my husband told me that he was mentally not ready to go to school. A year later, I paid for him to go. I worked two jobs and worked part-time in two other locations to make sure it happened. Two years later, I was so happy for him because he graduated! Then he said, "I do not feel like applying for a job in that field."

I don't think that it was wrong for me to make my husband and his dream a priority. What I did wrong was not taking the time to make myself and my own needs a priority. I was so focused on him that I forgot about myself. I got lost in the process. Enablers usually find themselves like this. All of their energy goes to the abuser.

If you don't take care of your needs to be loved, to feel secure, and to be happy, you can easily end up feeling frustrated, stressed out, depressed, resentful, or angry. This is not healthy. You have to protect yourself and work on your healing. (We will talk more about this in chapter 6.)

THE INABILITY TO DISPLAY EMOTION

Even though I knew their behavior was unacceptable, I did not feel hurt from the way my accountant or my employer treated me. It was probably because, over the years, my heartbreak had made me numb to the pain of the abuse in my marriage. This was how I tried to protect myself. I had learned to distance myself from my feelings. I had put up a shield around my heart. I did not want to allow new acquaintances to come too close anymore.

All the time when I was making excuses—not requiring my husband to be accountable, taking up his slack, not setting boundaries, not following through with any consequences, putting all of his needs first, not thinking about myself, and being defensive—I was pretending to be okay. I had a smile on my face, but inside I was cold and hollow. I found true love in my children. But the need to be loved as a woman had been pushed back somewhere and forgotten.

If you have gotten to the point where you are not able to show any emotion or even talk about how you feel about your abuse, your coldness and silence may be enabling the abuse to continue in your life. Don't continue to walk around like the living dead. You don't have to live like a zombie. Just like the Prophet Ezekiel asked the Spirit of God to breathe life into the valley of dry bones, you can ask the Holy Spirit to breathe life back into your soul.

YOUR DIVINE REFLECTION

The Best Lens

In your journal, write down the best lens (or scriptures) to look through in the Word of God so that you will be able to identify the behaviors of the abuser that you will not help to enable.

Here are four examples to get your started:

1. "Assume your own responsibility." Galatians 6:5 (GW)
2. "But if someone does not provide for his own, especially his own family, he has denied the (Christian) faith, and is worse than an unbeliever." 1 Timothy 5:8 (NET)
3. "The one who is unwilling to work shall not eat. We hear that some among you are idle and disruptive. They are not busy....Such people we command and urge in the Lord Jesus Christ to settle down and earn the food they eat...never tire in doing what is good. Take special note of anyone who does not obey our instruction in this letter. Do not associate with them, in order that they may feel ashamed." 2 Thessalonians 3:11-14 (NIV)
4. "Have nothing to do with the fruitless deeds of darkness, but rather expose them." Ephesians 5:11 (NIV)

The Big Picture

In your journal, write your own prayer to God that He will give you His eternal view of your marriage. Ask God to give you His wisdom to be able to set boundaries that are respectful and consequences that are protective for you.

Here is my prayer for you:

Father God, we thank You that You are a God of mercy and justice. Forgive us for missing the mark of not following Your Word as we should. Help us to not support an environment of wrong behavior and irresponsibility. Help my sister to not make excuses for her husband or get offended by the truth about herself. You said in Your Word that if we need wisdom to ask You for it, and that You would give it to us. I ask for Your wisdom for my sister right now. Give her what to say as she speaks the truth in love to her husband. Let her know what is just on her behalf. Give her the courage and strength to stand up for righteousness. Help her to love herself and stand for what is right for herself in accordance to how You want her to be cared for. Take away her stony heart and give her a heart that is tender and sensitive to You and others. In Jesus' name I pray. Amen.

Heart Vision

Close your eyes and look at your heart. What does it look and feel like? Does it look hard or soft? Does it feel cold or warm? Is it in pain, or is it healed? When you open your eyes, write in your journal what you saw.

1. Answer these questions in your journal:
2. You married because of love, but now do you feel that your husband's behavior has hurt you? In what way?
3. If I asked you whether YOU are a battered woman, would you immediately feel angry or offended? Why?
4. Are you making any excuses for why your husband is acting immature or not being responsible? If so, what are the excuses?

5. Are you constantly making your husband a priority, rather than yourself? In what ways?

6. Are there some boundaries that need to be put in place so that you will feel safe and secure? If so, what are they?

7. Are you ready to face the consequences of your husband's not wanting to adhere to your boundaries? Do you feel that you and your children are worth more than what you may have to sacrifice in order to have the life that you deserve?

Shine Your Light

After reading this chapter, you might have identified some ways that you have been enabling your husband's abusive behaviors. From now own, the blind spot of enabling will not be a hindrance, keeping you from standing up for yourself so that you will be respected.

In your journal, write six things that you can do this week to let your light shine and put your heart vision into motion.

Answer these questions in your journal:

1. What can you decide to ask for from your husband that will cause one or more major changes at home?

2. What are you going to do differently if your husband doesn't do what you asked?

3. When can you set an appointment to talk to one or both of you support persons that you identified in chapters 1 and 3? Make an appointment with a professional counselor if you feel you may be in danger. Talk with your support team about the boundaries and consequences that you want for yourself and ask your support person(s) to help you make a safe plan to ask for

a change that you want. Let them know that you need a plan in case you have to face negative consequences if your husband doesn't agree to your suggested change. Let one or both of your support people know when you are planning on talking to your husband.

4. When can you set a good time and in what safe public place (that you can drive to and from separately from your husband if necessary) can you go to discuss your boundaries with your husband and let him know what you will do if he does not agree to them? Let your husband know about your support person. If he dismisses what you have to say, let him know that you are sorry he feels that way, and leave. Ask your support person to either be there at your meeting place at a distance, to call to check on you every ten minutes, or allow you and your children to spend the night if necessary.

5. When can you set up a follow-up meeting with your support person(s) to make sure you are following through with your consequences?

6. What can you do to make yourself a priority this week?

E—Esteem

YOUR ESTEEM HELPS YOU SEE CLEARLY

I want to share with you a tale about a caterpillar's transformation (inspired by *A Butterfly that Thought It Was still a Caterpillar: A Transformation Story* from exploringyourmind. com published on Jan. 17, 2018).

> There was once a caterpillar who thought she was fat and ugly. For years, she inched along on her legs and admired all of the other beautiful animals and plants in the garden where she lived.

One day, she decided to climb a tall tree. It took her a long time to get to a high-enough branch so that she could see the whole garden in one view. She saw the beautiful flowers, the magnificence of the blue sky as the white clouds floated by, and the beautiful birds as they gracefully flew by.

And then out of nowhere she saw a swarm of beautiful butterflies. Oh, how she wished she were a butterfly! But she was nothing but a worm that crawled around in the dirt, ate leaves all day, and got fat. She had no friends or family. She felt as if she were all alone.

Over the last few weeks, her skin had been shedding over and over. This made her feel even worse about herself. She thought, "I look hideous." She started shedding again, but this time her skin looked different. It was more like silk, and it became sticky. It stuck on the branch of the tree. It felt so good that she decided to stay right there. The skin got hard and turned into a shell. She was so tired that she fell asleep for a long time.

She finally woke up. She was in a dark place and wanted to get out. She felt cramped and trapped. She could hardly move. She struggled and struggled to get out. Finally, the hard shell cracked. Out popped her head, then her body, and then a slimy liquid covered her body and flowed over a heavy weight that she now carried on her back.

Not realizing what had happened to her, she kept walking on her legs, but now it was very hard because she was carrying around such a heavy weight on her back. She stopped trying to put one foot in front of the other and became very sad. She did not know why she could not move forward anymore. She was so exhausted.

A beautiful blue butterfly flew over and landed next to her. He said, "Hi beautiful. What's wrong?"

She cried, "I can't climb this tree like I used to. My legs are too weak."

He asked, "Why don't you use your wings?" and then he fluttered away.

For the first time, she realized that she had wings. She stretched and opened them wide. They were beautiful and purple. She was no longer an ugly, fat caterpillar. She no longer had to crawl around on the ground like she did in the past. She was the most beautiful butterfly that she had ever seen. She realized how magnificent, wonderful, and unique she really was. The God of all creation had shined His light on her!

The problem was, she did not know how to fly. She had never done that before...But her wings were so pretty. She liked to open and close them just to admire them. Over and over, she kept saying to herself, "You are beautiful." She had never felt like this before. She became more confident in herself. She believed she could fly. "The sky is the limit!" she said.

A little at a time, as she kept flapping her beautiful, purple wings, she got stronger and stronger. The most exhilarating moment in her life was when she lifted her legs and took flight. Her perspective of the garden as she soared in the air was totally different from her past when she was a caterpillar crawling on the ground.

Before she got to the place where she trusted herself to fly, part of her wanted to experience her new life as a butterfly, and the other part of her wanted to continue to live in the past where she was comfortable. It took time to discover her strength after she felt good about herself. It took time to discover how to use her wings, and she realized that she needed help and encouragement.

Sometimes, you may not want to accept change (because you feel afraid, embarrassed, or inadequate) even when you have the power and ability to transform your life. You don't have to try to do it alone. Sometimes, others can see you better than you can see yourself.

In this chapter, we talk about how your opinion of yourself can affect your attitude and your decision to face change in your life much like the butterfly in our story. I will reveal how having low esteem can be a blind spot keeping you from navigating your path forward on your MAP to SEE.

THE IMPORTANCE OF SELF-IMAGE

I had the lowest self-image growing up as a preteen and teenager. Just like the caterpillar in the opening story of this chapter, I saw myself as fat and ugly. I kept to myself. I felt invisible. I was the homely, plain girl in the back of the classroom with pigtails, a long skirt, tennis shoes, no jewelry, and Vaseline on my lips—even throughout middle school. Now that was a tragedy for any tween girl.

My mom finally convinced my dad to let me curl my hair when I was in the ninth grade. I would sit at my mirror in my pink bedroom and look at the beautiful models in *Ebony* and *Jet* magazines. I dreamed that one day I would look pretty like them.

Because I was not one of the cute, popular girls like the cheerleaders or dancers on the drill team, I concentrated on my grades. My classmates elected me "Most Likely to Succeed." That boosted my self-image, but two weeks into my freshman year in college, the worst thing that I could image happened. I lost the only part of me that I thought was pretty. All of my hair fell out!

I was staying in Crosby Hall, which was a freshman female dorm at Ole Miss. One night, I went down the hallway to the common bathroom. When I passed the mirror, I saw how limp my hair looked. I went over to the sink and ran my hand through my hair. As I did my dry, brittle hair from the right side of my head fell down into the sink. I gasped in panic. The same thing happened to my hair on the left side.

Within a few minutes, I ended up with a few strands of hair sticking out of the top of my head. I looked like a chicken! I started crying hysterically. I remembered that the day before, I had gotten a perm in my hair. The beautician had left the chemicals in my hair too long. My hair was over processed. I did not know how I could bare to face the world on my college campus the next day. I still wore the long skirts, tennis shoes, no jewelry, and Vaseline on my lips. I wore the ugliest glasses, and now I was bald.

I put on a baseball cap and wore it every day for several years. I kept to myself. I went to my classes and came back to my dorm room each day as quickly as possible. I wanted to disappear. I still felt invisible.

I did not realize how much my poor self-image affected my

behavior. Your self-image can affect what you do (and don't do). How you perceive yourself can affect where you go (and don't go). It affects who you associate with (and who you don't). It took me a while to learn this valuable lesson as I went through my life's journey.

How much other people value you can sometimes be a reflection of how much you value yourself. How much other people respect you can sometimes be a reflection of how much you respect yourself. If you don't think other people should do special things to honor you, you will miss your blessing. You will reject the fact that you deserve to be treated like the magnificent, wonderful, unique woman of God that your Father God created. When He created you, the Word of God said you were wonderfully and beautifully made. Girlfriend, you have to know who you are!

WHO ARE YOU?

In the Disney film, *The Lion King*, Mufasa had to remind his son, Simba, that he was the royal heir to the throne. With the same words, I am here to tell you to "remember who you are."

As I mentioned in chapter 4, I believe that you are a spirit. You have a soul, and you live in a body. The Word of God says that God is the Father of spirits. Therefore, you can say that God created your spirit, which is the real you on the inside. I believe that your spirit lives in the housing of your body. Your body looks the way it does because you got your physical genetic traits from a mother and a natural father.

The Word of God says that God is the King of Kings. That means He is the King over all the other kings. The Word of God also says that He makes us kings (and queens). So, in the spiritual realm, other spiritual beings (angels and demonic spirits) recognize the children of God as royalty. God, being the King, has a kingdom. He reigns over everything in His heavenly kingdom. Another word for heaven and His heavenly kingdom is *Zion*. So, God reigns over Zion.

The Word of God says that if you are a part of his family, you are a part of His royal priesthood. Kings and priests are who we are. When you become a believer and accept Jesus as your Lord and savior of your life, He makes your spirit in right standing with Him. We are the Righteousness of God, in Christ Jesus. God adopts you into His spiritual family. (See appendix C if you want to be adopted by God.) When God adopts you, something miraculous happens.

Just like the butterfly goes through a metamorphosis and a new creature is created, the same thing happens to your spirit. A new spirit is created that has spiritual traits like your Father God. As I mentioned in chapter 1, these spiritual traits are referred to as the "fruit of the Spirit" and is given to you by the Holy Spirit. You can call Him Father God, because He is your spiritual father. He is the father of your new, recreated spirit.

SARAH'S DAUGHTER

In the Old Testament (part 1) of the Bible, God made a promise to a man named Abraham. His wife was named Sarah. Abraham and Sarah were very rich and were part of the royal nobility of their day. They were wealthy with lots of land, cattle, and servants. God told Abraham that he was going to be the father of many nations. So, his sons would be rulers of many tribes and nations. Abraham's children became the children of Israel. They came to be known as God's chosen people.

In the New Testament (part 2) of the Bible, Jesus gave the world a new promise—we ALL can be a part of the family of God. Just like all of God's children can call him Father God, the Bible says that we can all call Abraham Father Abraham. This is because all of God's children are still considered the spiritual seeds of Abraham.

I remember singing the Father Abraham song that many children learn in Sunday school. The lyrics to the main verse are:

"Father Abraham had many sons,
Many sons had Father Abraham,
I am one of them and so are you,
So, let's all praise the Lord."

Well, my question is: "What about the daughters?" I know that in the Bible, many times when the male gender is brought up, it is just *understood* that females are included, too. But little girls singing this song and women who don't know to use inferences need to be told, "You are the Daughters of Sarah."

As I mentioned in chapter 1, some years ago I would go to my godmother's house for a monthly women's bible study in her beautiful home. One sunny, Saturday morning, Ms. Willa gave the ladies a declaration of who we are spiritually. She told us to say it out loud so that we could hear ourselves. This is what we boldly said in unison:

"We are descended from the aristocracy of the Lord—
From a higher and nobler race that even Gentile Kings may boast;
A privilege and glory of which
no circumstance, no affliction, no persecution

can deprive us—
Ours,
through all and every event of life, unless we cast it from us,
Forsaking for ambition or gold, or power,
the banner of our blessed faith.
We cannot be deprived of our birthright,
Unless like Esau, we exchange it for worldly riches or grati-
fication.
We are Sarah's daughters,
The chosen, the beloved of the Lord!"

Sarah was a woman of nobility, a woman of grace and excellence. If she is your spiritual mother, *your spirit* should reflect a spirit of grace and excellence. You, as a woman of God, are a Daughter of Zion. We are God's daughters in His heavenly kingdom. God is also a God of grace and excellence. We have His spiritual DNA.

God has given His daughters a spirit of power, love, and a strong mind. Queens and princesses are who we are. You have to know who you are when you walk in the room. You deserve honor and respect because of where God has placed you in the Kingdom of God.

DON'T BE ROBBED OF WHO YOU ARE

The experience of actually discovering that I did not know what I liked or what I wanted in my life for myself anymore was one of the most embarrassing moments of my life. Let me tell you how it happened.

In 2003, we had a guest speaker, Peter Daniels, come to Word of Faith Christian Center in Jackson, Mississippi. He is the author of the book, *How to Reach Your Life Goals*. During his presentation, he had time for audience participation.

He asked, "Can I get five volunteers to help me explain the concept of setting goals?"

"Well," I thought to myself, "this is easy. I have always been a goal setter. I have set goals in the past to have a family, a higher education, and a professional career."

So, I raised my hand. Out of the five hundred people in the congregation in attendance, I was one of the five people he chose. I excitedly walked down the aisle and stood on the stage to the far left of the podium. I was the last one on the end. He pointed to a chart that read "One-Year, Five-Year, and Ten-Year Goals."

He asked the five of us, "Within one of these time periods, if you could have anything in the world, tell me three things that you desire. The sky is the limit."

My other four church members quickly rattled off huge sums of money and elaborate material desires that sounded great. And then he came to me.

He asked me, "What are three things that you desire?"

I wanted to sound great too, so I said, "Money!"

He chimed in and asked, "How much?"

I had never set a certain amount of money to be my goal, so I just said an excessive figure like the others had.

"A half a billion dollars," I said off the top of my head.

He said, "Okay, and what are the other two?"

I thought to myself, "If I had that much money, I would not need to name any other material things because I could buy anything else that I may want in the future."

So, I was at a loss for words. I knew what my husband would want. He would want a million-dollar estate home. I had walked through many with him as he imagined our family living in one. He would want a luxury car. I had sat in our old car many a time as he walked through car lots at night after hours with dreamy eyes. He would want expensive jewelry. He would get watches and rings from pawn shops and thrift stores quite often.

But none of those things were my dreams. I had stopped dreaming of having my own optometry practice. That did not even come up in my spirit. So, I did not even think about that. But I did want to serve God in the ministry in some way. I did not know what area.

I spoke up and said, "I want a ministry service to devote my life to."

He said, "No. That is not a tangible goal. What we are discussing here are tangible objects that you can touch and feel. Not intangible things like service, a career, and relationships. What is an object that is concrete that you desire, that would be valuable to you to work toward as a prize?"

I had nothing. I did not have anything on the inside that I wanted. In that moment in front of everybody, I was located. I realized that I did not have a tangible dream for myself. I did not have anything in my heart that was "for me."

I had been so engrossed in what my husband wanted to make him happy that I had forgotten about me. So, there I stood in front of the whole church with a blank stare on my face. There was total silence in the church. Every eye was on me.

I just looked at him. He looked back at me, and he finally broke the deafening silence with, "I'm waiting, and I'm not moving on until you tell me something that you want."

I started to get hot. My hands started to sweat. My eyes started to well up with tears, but I fought them back. I stood there for what seemed like an eternity.

Peter Daniels eventually said, "This is not unusual. So many people don't have a dream for themselves."

Church members started shouting out things for me to say as if I were on a game show. One person shouted out, "A new car!" Someone else screamed, "A new house!" and another person tried to help me by shouting out, "A 10-carat diamond ring!"

The problem was that those things were not my dreams. I had already blurted out a huge sum of money, even though that was not my dream, either. It had just sounded good when the others said it. In order to get out of the hot seat, I said, "A plane and a multimillion-dollar property of personal real estate." Again, I just pulled something out of the air.

Peter Daniels looked at each of the volunteers and pointed back to the chart that he had on display. He said, "Because of this time table, you have all set goals that are virtually impossible. Given where you may be now and where you want to go in a certain amount of time, you could not get there. Goals have to be specific, realistic, and reachable. This day will be a mark on your lives to dream and set realistic goals. You all can take your seats."

As I slowly walked back to my seat, I was not only embarrassed, I was challenged. I went home and with tears running down my face, I asked God for my own dream. I wanted a vision of an image for my eyes of faith to focus on so that I could create something beautiful and tangible in my life that I could see in the natural and say, "It is good."

That day was definitely a mark on my life. I did not have practice at creating. I did not have a "let there be" goal to create something physical as God had. He found pleasure as He saw His physical creations because they were good.

Because I did not have a tangible dream, I did not have a

vision for it. I had not allowed myself to take a glimpse into God's bounty to see what He had in store for me. I had not looked into the spiritual realm, which is where the things in this physical world come from. Everything tangible that you see starts with someone having a dream of it. Then he or she creates it.

I needed practice using my spiritual vision. What had God put in my heart to see? When I closed my eyes that night, I saw an image of my own optometry practice. There it was, just like I had shared with my dad years ago. For the last few years before that night, I had not seen myself as a strong, influential business owner. I saw myself only as a weary mother of two small children, struggling to work at any clinic that needed fill-in help so that I could keep my family together and my husband from being upset. I was not living my life by faith. I was living my life by my eyesight.

Everything wrong that was going on in my personal life, I saw as a reflection of me. I did not see myself as worthy or capable. I had only negative labels for myself. "I was not pretty," was one of these thoughts. I had a long history of telling myself that. My husband never told me that I was pretty. I guess, subconsciously, because he did not affirm that I was beautiful, it just confirmed that I was not—at least to him.

We were struggling financially. I had to make sure my children were taken care of at every turn. I thought that my husband spent way too much money on excessive clothes, shoes, and jewelry for himself. So, I dared not spend any money on myself (other than keeping my hair styled). As I mentioned earlier, my hair had fallen out when I was in college. I did not want anything like that to happen again. I figured taking care of my hair was a necessity because of my profession. I did not feel like I had enough time in a day to juggle all the challenges of work, home, church, motherhood, and a destructive marriage.

My self-esteem was so low that I had lost connection with myself. What I wanted was no longer important. What my husband liked and wanted was important to me. I did not put a value on my wants and desires. My whole world centered on trying to keep my family afloat. I worked long hours trying to pay all the bills. I had to spend more time than average with my children on their homework. I took them to all extracurricular activities. I made church twice a week a priority. I was a praying wife.

I remember praying so many times, "God, help me to know how to please my husband." And that is a good prayer to pray as a wife. However, it is not a good prayer when you are in a destructive marriage and your husband will never truly be content. When your husband is not happy on the inside, praying that you can somehow change or do something different that will make him happy will not work because nothing that you can do will make him happy. The love, peace, and blessing that your husband needs has to come from God. *Your husband has to be willing to be in agreement with what God wants him to do before he can be in agreement with what you want him to be.*

I did not have any personal passion in life to live for myself. My only passion was my relationship with the Lord. Have you ever felt like you had no passion for yourself? Do you feel like you don't have a physical goal to work toward? That you don't have a wish for yourself that you can sink your teeth into?

It is time for you to start looking with your heart. Ask God to give you a vision for yourself so that you will not perish. You should not be walking around like a zombie, as if you are the living dead. The Word of God says that "without a vision, My people perish." Don't allow yourself to be so overly involved with someone else that you lose yourself in the process. Don't be robbed of who you are.

RESTORING WHO YOU ARE

I had to find out my value in God's eyes. The Word of God says that I am the apple of His eye. Jesus said that the second-most important Commandment in the Bible was that we love our neighbors as ourselves. Yes, we must love others, but also, we must love ourselves.

After I moved back to my home state of Mississippi and got a divorce, I remember one counseling session with my pastor. He told me, "Dellia, you deserve to be cared for and nurtured and treated with deep affection because you are extremely special to God. The Bible says, 'to Him, your worth is far above the value of jewels.'"

When he told me that, I started crying so hard that I could not compose myself. It was as if something had broken lose and been released on the inside of my heart. I needed to hear those words of life to start my healing process.

In that moment, I also remembered what my godmother, Ms. Willa, had told me seven years before. She had said, "Dellia, you are Father God's precious daughter. You are the King's daughter. God does not want His daughter to be treated wrong. You deserve to be treated like royalty, because that is what the Word says who you are."

I had to love myself the same way God loved me. I had to see myself as God saw me. It was so easy for me to love others, but it was hard for me to love Dellia as much. I had to learn that I could love someone, but I did not have to let the person I loved disrespect me because I knew my value. I was worth more than that.

I got my inspiration from a beautiful, strong, courageous woman in the Bible named Queen Esther who had a makeover with months of beauty treatments. Her makeover included skin treatments, oils, perfumes, and cosmetics. You already know that her attire must have also been on point.

Pampering myself gave me the confidence that I needed to accomplish my goals. After my divorce, I made friends with a hair stylist, a nail tech, a Mary Kay director, a personal trainer, and a massage therapist. They were all part of my support team. I kept appointments with them regularly. My fashion-savvy friends took me shopping for some different clothes and cute shoes.

Low and behold, I was asked to go out on a date. That was a little scary because I had been out of the dating scene for twenty years. I rallied my support team. I got all dolled up. I looked at myself in the mirror, and I was surprised at what I saw. I said, "I look beautiful," just like the butterfly in the story at the beginning of this chapter.

When I actually went on this date, as my date and I entered the restaurant, another guy sitting at another table with his date told me, "You look stunning!" Well, that was a first. But the thing about it was, for the first time, I actually believed it. I thought that I looked beautiful and I felt amazing. That feeling of confidence in myself motivated me to do amazing things. I knew because of scripture that I could do all things through Christ who strengthened me. But, when I felt good about myself, I was more encouraged to do all of those things.

I had to schedule time to celebrate myself and what I enjoyed. Besides scheduling appointments to pamper myself, I set aside time to go places by myself and with friends to the movies, out to eat, and weekend girls' trips. I set aside time to read interesting books, do scrapbooking, and enjoy bubble baths with candles and instrumental music.

You have to reconnect with yourself to find out what you truly like. You have to rediscover what you want and do not want. You have to look with your spiritual eyes to see who you are. You have to choose to make yourself a priority and not allow someone else to dominate your existence.

You are royalty and have a spirit of excellence. You are beautiful, strong, and competent. Don't listen to the lies that the enemy whispers in your ear, saying, "No one else will love you. You won't find anyone else better. You are being selfish. You are not worthy." He told me the same ones....But let me tell you this one thing, "The Devil is a lie!" The word of God says that he is the father of lies in John 8:44.

The sky is the limit to what you can do in life and what God can do through your life. Love yourself first. Be content with yourself first. Love the skin you are in. Do what you can. Leave the rest to God. Spread your beautiful wings so that you can soar. Make it a habit of treating yourself. You deserve it. This is not being selfish. This is just loving yourself.

YOUR DIVINE REFLECTION

The Best Lens

In your journal, write down the best lens (or scriptures) to look through in the Word of God so that low esteem will not cause you to have a distorted view of who you actually are and what God wants you to do.

Here are four examples to get you started:

1. "And You have made us (God's children) kings (and queens), and priests to our God; And we shall reign on the earth." Revelations 5:10 NKJV

2. Jesus answered him, "Love the Lord your God with all your heart, with all your soul, and with all your mind. This is the greatest and most important commandment." The Second Commandment is similar to it: "Love your neighbor as you **love yourself.**" Matthew 37-39 GNT

3. "Where there is no vision, the people perish." Proverbs 29:18a KJV

4. "She had to complete twelve months of beauty treatments prescribed for the women, six months with oil of myrrh and six with perfumes and cosmetics." Esther 2:12b NIV

The Big Picture

In your journal, write your own prayer to God that He will give you His eternal view of yourself. Ask Him to help you see yourself like He sees you.

Here is my prayer for you:

Father God, You are Elohim, the God that creates. Thank

You for creating our spirits and creating us in your image. Thank You that in Your kingdom our rank is right under the angels.

Thank You for adopting us in Your kingdom when we believe in Your Son, Jesus. Thank You for making us a part of Your royal priesthood. I pray for my sister that she agrees with Your Word that You made her wonderful and beautiful.

As a believer, I pray she receives the revelation that she is Your daughter and a daughter of Zion. I pray that as she understands her spirit of nobility and excellence, she will with confidence walk in her authority as a daughter of Sarah. And then help her not to throw away her confidence.

Thank You for giving her the spirit of love, power, and a strong mind. Help her to be Godly, proud of herself, and to believe in herself. Be the lifter of her head.

Help her to love, stand up for, and look out for herself. Help her to be strong and courageous. Give her the courage to make the right decisions that will bring needed change in her life and in the lives of her children. Lead her to the right people who will be an advocate for her. Protect her from all hurt, harm, and danger. All these things I ask in your Son Jesus' name. Amen

Heart Vision

Close your eyes and in your heart see how you would look if you were given a makeover that was fit for a queen. How would your hair, makeup, clothes, shoes, and accessories look? When you open your eyes, describe how you saw yourself.

Answer these questions in your journal:

1. What scented candles, oils, perfumes, and lotions do you like?
2. Because you are a daughter of Sarah with a spirit of excellence, beauty and order, what changes would you like to make in your living quarters?
3. What tangible dream do you have in your heart for yourself?

Shining Your Light

After reading and reflecting on this chapter, I believe your self-confidence will continue to grow. I hope that *not* believing in yourself will *no longer* be the blind spot that holds you back from what God wants you to do. He wants you to be true to yourself. He wants you to take care of yourself and your children so that your lives will truly glorify Him.

In your journal, write four things that you can do this week to let your light shine and put your heart vision into motion.

Answer these questions and do these assignments in your journal:

- What can you do to make a step toward bringing to reality the tangible dream that you wrote down in your heart vision exercise?
- Write two lists: one of the things you like about yourself, and another of the things you want for yourself.
- What are you going to clean and put in order to make your living quarters fit for a queen?
- What are you going to do to pamper yourself?

CHAPTER 7

Moving Forward to Your Purpose

As I mentioned in chapter 1, six years before I left my husband, I had fled another state, Alabama, on the run, trying to get away from him after he had threatened my life. I physically moved to Mississippi, but I did not move forward with my life because *I was not ready.*

I was convinced that he was going to change, and I was going to be the one to help him. I was not aware of the term *domestic violence*. I did not think of myself as a victim. I did not know the signs of emotional, verbal, financial, or physical abuse in intimate relationships even though I was experiencing symptoms of each one.

I also explained how my home was no longer a safe place to live for me and my children. Even though I had the locks changed on our house, I was still afraid to go back there because of his threatening messages, vandalizing of property, and his stalking me despite having a restraining order. My attorney said that at the end of the day, the restraining order was only a piece of paper. She made me aware that my marriage had the hallmark signs of a typical abusive marriage. She advised me that I needed to leave the state immediately for my safety.

I called one of my sisters-in-law in Jackson and asked her to book a flight for me the next day. I hired two off-duty police officers to come to the house while my husband was at work. I had them stand guard while a moving company that I hired packed up our belongings. I left the new keys to the house so that my husband could reassume residency. When I walked out of my house that day, *I was finally ready to move on.*

No one can make up your mind for you. *You have to be ready to move forward when you know the uncertainty of leaving is far better than the insecurity of staying.* You have to look inside your heart and see what your heart wants. Ask God for direction, and let your spirit lead you.

RECALCULATING

There were several trips that I had to make back and forth from Tulsa to Jackson all by myself. That was a little daunting, but thank goodness I had my GPS. All I needed to have was the address of my destination and look for convenient gas stations along the way. When I got off the interstate, the GPS would recalculate my trip, and I would move forward without a problem.

In a similar fashion, I had to turn on my spiritual GPS of the Holy Spirit to navigate how to move forward with my new life as I made the transition from being married for twenty years to being single again. My original plan for my life was to get married, have a loving home, have children, and live happily ever after. Sound familiar? When I got a divorce, my life's vision was lost.

God knew in His sovereign plan for my life that I had to get my vision lined up with His vision for my life. By getting a divorce, this was the only way for me to put the past in the past. I could not hold onto my old way of doing things and still move forward. I had to press forward to the new thing that He wanted me to do in my life.

After I first asked God, "What do I do next?" I kept asking Him that same question over and over. We have our plans, but God directs our steps. I had to pray for God to let me see His perspective for my life. I had to be open to where the Holy Spirit was leading me because now, I was following God's vision and not mine. After not having a car, I was happy to drive an old hooptie that was given to me. I worked on four different part-time jobs at one time – seven days a week — before I purchased my practice.

I looked at a lot of homes in different cities and was still searching for a mortgage when I moved into my home. I socialized with other men whom God did not lead me into lasting relationships with before I met the man God meant for me and remarried.

As I moved along in my life, I kept asking God, "What do I do next?" But I had to make the choices and do the moving. As

I listened to the voice of the Holy Spirit, confessed God's word that He would give me wisdom, and heeded godly counsel, I was willing and obedient to the Holy Spirit's rerouting of my direction. I trusted that God knew what was best for me. I had to trust in my relationship with God to get me to a better place that I could not see.

As a believer, once you have followed the guidelines that I mentioned above, you can move forward with confidence knowing that God is in control of your path in life. You should not be afraid to make a decision as long as you stay within these parameters. Even if you take a detour, trust God to reroute you back on your path. Don't be so afraid to move that you don't move at all. I once heard one of my coaches tell me, "You can't move a parked car." So, come on and move out of park and pass neutral. It's time for you to drive.

LESSON LEARNED

My two children are both adults now. I am so proud to be their mom. During their high school years, they both exhibited those sometimes-difficult teen stages. They both made "smart" comments to me and wanted to exercise their independence and see how far they could bend the rules of the house.

My daughter is older, so she decided to challenge me and the house rules first. Two years later, my son decided to do the same. I told both of them the same things, "I love you, but I will not allow you to disrespect me. If you cannot be respectful, you will have to find somewhere else to live." I had learned my lesson.

Of course, I did not want them to leave. They had to make their own decisions, and I am glad that they both decided to stay. But I had to stand up for myself and let the chips fall where they may. Otherwise, they would not have respected me, and I would have felt that they had taken advantage of me.

Part of moving forward in your life is learning from your life lessons. You have to stand in your authority to make your own choices because of the free will that God gives you. Continue to set boundaries for yourself and follow through with consequences. This is part of every healthy relationship.

FORGIVENESS

Going through the process of forgiveness was the only way for me to move forward. Until I was able to extend forgiveness, I was stuck. Forgiveness helped to pry loose the tight grip of bitterness and resentment that my heart was holding onto. In my own strength and ability, I could not forgive my ex-husband. I had to feel and work through the pain that I had wanted to be numb to for so long. I did not want to talk about or acknowledge or even remember the pain. But I had to remember it in order to forgive it. I had to release my anger by throwing my hurt off me to rest at the feet of Jesus.

I did not feel any different. Forgiveness is not a feeling; it is a choice. When I closed my eyes, when I thought about my ex-husband in my heart, I saw myself back in the darkness of that night when I left him. But the roles were now reversed. Instead of seeing him having our daughter pinned on the ground, in my spirit, I saw myself having him pinned down with my hands around his thick neck.

In my spirit, I had to make a choice to release him from my clutches. I had to take my hands off his neck. But I could not do it on my own. Despite the many prayers I said that I forgave him, I still harbored the pain of his hurting me emotionally, physically, and verbally; not taking care of me on so many levels; disappointing me; betraying me; not loving me or being there for me like he had promised to.

Because he has a soul just like me that needs grace and mercy, I made a choice to forgive him by rejecting negative thoughts and praying positive words. I knew that if I did not stop holding him accountable for hurting me, God would not stop holding me accountable for my desire to put him in a sleeper hold every time I thought about his abusive behaviors toward me and our children.

I had to put my trust in the Holy Spirit to supernaturally remove the stronghold of resentment and bitterness. Forgiving my ex-husband did not mean that he should not show integrity and do the right thing and be accountable. It just meant that I was rolling his offenses over to God, and I was not going to hold hurtful feelings and thoughts against him in my heart.

I could not do it on my own. It was not until I started praying for him and his life, salvation, and well-being that I could close my eyes, and in my heart, see him released from my trying to harm him and walking toward God in the light of dawn. You see, I had to release him to God. I had to let God be the one to deal with him with His eternal love and justice.

A few years ago, I wrote him a letter letting him know that I had chosen to let go of holding a grudge, and I sent him a gift card. Sending him money did not make sense to me at first when the Holy Spirit told me to do it one morning during my quiet time that I was spending with God.

I was thinking to myself, "Are you crazy? Have you forgotten all of the money and stuff that he has taken from you over the years? Even now, he is denying that he owes back child support. You know your children are in college. You have bills to pay."

And the negative thoughts kept coming and coming. I had to resist the impulse to want to get back at him. I had to respond to those thoughts with grace and mercy.

I had to apply Matthew 5:44 that says that you should pray for and do good to them that despitefully use you. I had to do something that was good for him. I had to be a doer of the Word of God and not only a hearer of the Word of God.

It was not a choice I could make only once to extend grace and mercy to my ex-husband that freed me once and for all. It is a choice that I have to make every day. I choose to think good thoughts. The Word of God says that we should think about whatever is good, pure, and worthy of praise. (Philippians 4:8) However, whenever I do get negative thoughts about my ex-husband, I decide not to let those thoughts enter my emotions.

I quickly say to myself, "Because of God's love, I choose to keep no record of wrongs, I choose to forgive him, and I pray that grace and mercy follow him all the days of his life." I make a conscience effort not to talk negatively about those thoughts and ask the Holy Spirit to help me continue to be a giver of grace and advocate for mercy.

GRACE AND MERCY

I am empowered to give mercy because God provides all of us mercy each morning. According to Lamentations 3:22-23, God's love for us is so great, and He is so faithful and just, that He gives us new mercy every morning.

This scripture is always such a blessing to me. Because of this scripture, I just want to give God a shout out of praise and say, "Hallelujah!" and do my church dance because whoever the Lord has set free is free indeed!

Let me share with you why I always rejoice in the Lord because of this scripture. Before I understood and applied this biblical principle, several years had gone by where I felt defeated and still could not forgive my ex-husband. I would say to God in prayer, "Lord, I forgive my ex-husband. I thank you that my heart is right with you, in Jesus' name. Amen." Then I would go about my life as usual. I would feel good for a while. Then something would be said, or something would trigger a memory of how my ex-husband had wronged me. I would immediately respond, on the defensive, from that dark place in my heart. I would get angry and upset all over again. My heart would not be in the right place. I would be disappointed with myself and ask God to forgive me and tell God again that I forgave my ex-husband. But I also had to learn how to forgive myself.

Sometimes, I wouldn't get riled up anymore over the things that used to get me angry, and I would think I was making progress, but something else would pop up, and my heart would not be in the right place again. And the cycle—of prayer then offense and prayer then offense—kept happening over and over. I was really discouraged about this.

I asked God what I was doing wrong. Again, during my personal quiet time with God, the Holy Spirit led me to Proverbs 24:16 that identifies what the life of a righteous person looks like. It says that those who are righteous, the children of God, may fall seven times, but they shall rise again.

Even though you may be His child, God knows in your humanness that you will need His grace and mercy to remain in fellowship with Him. And because of His great love for you and His faithfulness, He makes mercy available for you to receive when you ask for it anew each morning.

You ask for His mercy because you are His child, you love

Him, and because you want to be in fellowship with Him. The only way that you can be in fellowship with Him is by being holy, which means your heart has to be pure and full of His light and not dark and full of evil desires.

In order to continue to be in a relationship with God, you cannot continue to harbor unforgiveness in your heart. (If you are a child of God, and for some reason you are not in fellowship with Him right now, and you want to get back in fellowship with Him, you can say the simple prayer in appendix C to get back in fellowship with God.)

If you do not want to be God's child, you will not have the desire to be in fellowship with Him. That is why the last part of that same scripture in Proverbs says that those who are not righteous will just stumble. They will not rise again because they are not even trying to maintain a relationship with God.

Now I hope you understand what it looks like to be one of the righteous children of God. When you receive His love, faithfulness, and mercy, you can give it to yourself and others who need it. Hopefully by doing this, you will not fall as much as you may have before you started the process of forgiveness. But when you do, He will be right there to pick you up when you call on Him because He promises to never leave you or forsake you. Until you go through this process of forgiveness, you cannot move forward toward your purpose in life. You will stay stuck.

YOUR PURPOSE

God put into motion my purpose in life the day I was born when my dad named me Dellia. Fast-forward thirty-five years later in April of 2004. I was attending a Discover Your Spiritual Destiny seminar one Saturday at church. The seminar was led by Dr. J. Victor and Catherine B. Eagan, coauthors of the book, *How to Discover Your Purpose in 10 Days*. While in one of the sessions, I remember asking God, "What do you want me to do with my life? Is there something else you want me to do?"

Three months later while working in an eye clinic in Jackson, God answered these questions. That was the day I mentioned in the introduction of this book when I heard God tell me that I was "His" optometrist, the one that He would use to help people see clearer with their spiritual eyes.

At that time, I had been practicing as an eye doctor for ten years, but that was the moment that I first had a glimpse of my true purpose in life. At that moment, I realized that I was equipped to apply the natural principles of optics that I had learned about how the eyes worked to the spiritual realm to help others be more aware of how they could use their faith. But this was just part of my revelation.

It was five years later in February of 2009 as I stood in a bookstore in Tulsa when I found out my full purpose was ordained by God from the day I was born. You see, I was always interested in finding the meaning of my name. I could never find my name on souvenir car tags or key chains. I knew that my name, Dellia, was a family name. My dad told me that he wanted to keep the name in the family because he had a sister named Dellia who had died as a week-old infant in the 1920s. But unbeknown to my dad, that was not the only reason God wanted me to be named Dellia.

I finally found my name's meaning in *The Name Book* by Dorothy Astoria that Saturday morning in the Mardel bookstore. I read in that book that Dellia means *visible. Visible* means "*to be able to see.*" Well, I had been working at that point for fifteen years helping people to do just that, to be able to see. *The Name Book* also gives the spiritual significance of each name. The spiritual meaning of *Dellia* is *divine reflection*. When I read that, I remembered what God had said to me five years earlier, that I was His spiritual eye doctor.

I told this story to one of my patients recently, and he said, "Wow, that is a great story! So, you being an optometrist was just meant to be." But I want to take that a step further and say, "I believe my purpose in life is to be what I like to call myself, 'God's optometrist.'"

Being an optometrist is not my purpose, but it has equipped and prepared me to fulfill my purpose of encouraging you to use your spiritual eyes to see what God wants to show you in your life. The tests and trials that I went through during and after my experience in an abusive relationship also helped prepare me to help others going through similar situations to reflect God's image in their lives. The Bible says that God made man in His own image. Because God is a spirit, He is talking about spiritually.

God's image is not of a person who is weak, insecure, fearful, ashamed, or defeated. God's image is of a person who is strong, courageous, confident, and victorious. This is what He wants for you. The decisions that you make will determine how and when you receive His promises to you.

I encourage you to depend on your spiritual sight when things don't look good to your natural eyesight. Trust in God to give you assurance and have faith in Him to guide you. When your faith is tested, your endurance gets stronger. Spiritually, you begin to grow when you depend on God. You begin to see God's supernatural ability is far greater than your limitations. You stop complaining. You stop crying. You stand up and square your shoulders. You realize who you are, and who God is in your life.

Your vocation is not your purpose. The position that you serve in church may not even be your life's purpose. *Your purpose is revealed when God suddenly shows up in your life and uniquely empowers you to help others like no one else can.* Your purpose is not given to lift you up on a pedestal. It is given to help others. It is given to glorify God. God shows up and deals in different ways with different people.

Sometimes, your purpose is what arouses compassion in you. Sometimes, it is what makes you angry or it is something you have a conviction about. Or, it might be the very thing that God has delivered you from so that you can help others in similar situations. This is how God gets the praise and glory from your life.

Your purpose might come easily to you, and you can do it exceptionally well. Or, it could be what you have a tendency to shy away from. Ask God why you feel this way. What dream do you have in your heart? The Holy Spirit will give you spiritual gifts that equip you for your purpose. What you go through on your life path prepares you for your purpose. Ask God to reveal your true purpose to you. Being bound and oppressed in an abusive relationship can hinder you from fulfilling your purpose.

The same blind spots that may cause you to not make a decision to move forward from an abusive relationship can also keep you from fulfilling your purpose. Unforgiveness, along with misunderstanding scriptures, anxieties, your and others' perceptions, not following your spirit, enabling and not setting boundaries, or low self-esteem can all hold you back from accomplishing your destiny.

But since I have made these blind spots *visible* to you, you can make the adjustments that are needed in order to make your dreams a reality. Hopefully, you are in a different place in your journey after using this MAP to SEE the reality of your situation better. When you know what you need to change, you can be true to yourself.

Now that you realize where you are, are you in a dark place? Do you want to move forward? After looking in your heart, searching the Word of God, praying and listening to God, and seeking godly counsel—ask yourself if you are in the place where God wants you to be. Are you ready to make a decision to change your life?

If you answered yes, you don't have to do this alone. Seek the help of a trusted friend, family member, or coworker. Get professional advice. Get help from legal offices with women's services, the police, government agencies, a women's shelter, or community associations that advocate for healthy and safe families. With their help, if you decide to leave an abusive relationship, put together a safe plan and transition into an independent home for yourself and your children.

As you trust in God, I believe that the Holy Spirit will light up your next step so that you can see clearly each turn that you should make. I believe that He will favor you with the right people across your path to provide exactly what you need at the right time. I believe that the power of the Holy Spirit will continue to strengthen you to carry out your calling.

Move forward expecting God to be God in your life. Close your eyes and look in your heart with the eyes of your faith. Fix your spiritual eyes on what you want God to create in your life. Use your authority to exercise your free will to make a decision to bring change.

Ask God for direction. Be sensitive to the Holy Spirit. Wait on the Lord in prayer during your devotional time, then get off your knees and do what you are led to do. Remember, faith without works is dead. I thank God with you in advance for bringing you to your place of safety and peace. And for this, let us give Him all the praise, honor, and glory!

YOUR DIVINE REFLECTION

The Best Lens

In your journal, write down the best lens (or scriptures) to look through the Word of God so that you will move forward with your life purpose.

Here are four examples to get you started:

1. "A person plans his way, but the Lord directs his steps." Proverb 16:9 (ISV)
2. "And my God will meet all your needs according to the riches of His glory in Christ Jesus." Philippians 4:19 (NIV)
3. "If you forgive men when they sin against you, your heavenly Father will also forgive you. But if you do not forgive men their sins, your Father will not forgive your sins." Matthew 6:14-15 (NLT)
4. "But I have raised you up for this very purpose, that I might show you My power and that My name might be proclaimed in all the earth." Exodus 9:16 (NIV)

The Big Picture

In your journal, write your own prayer to God that He will help you to forgive yourself and your abuser and give you His eternal view of your path forward toward your purpose.

Here is a prayer that you can pray to forgive your abuser:

Father God, thank You for being the God who sees. Thank You for being so good to me. Thank You for caring so much about me and how my heart has been hurt. You know the pain that I have felt because of (tell God the reasons for all of the pain and hurt that you have). Right now, I release and cast all of this hurt and pain at your feet, God.

Thank You, Jesus for dying on the cross for my sins, and I make a choice to forgive (his name) as an act of my free will. I reject all thoughts of revenge for (his name). I release my right to hold him accountable to me. I trust You, God that in Your own time and way, You will take care of (his name) according to Your will. Thank You, Holy Spirit for giving me Your power to forgive so that I can have freedom. All of these things I ask in Jesus' name. Amen.

Here is my prayer for you:

Father God, I thank You that You are Love. You are faithful, just, and full of mercy. As my sister seeks You on the direction she is to take in her life, I thank You that You order her steps. Thank You for being the Lord who is her shepherd. Because You are her Shepherd, You lead and guide her. I thank You that she shall not want any good thing, because You will give her what she desires, and help her to be content.

Thank You for supplying the finances and material needs that she needs for herself and her children while she goes through this time in her life. Connect her with the right people at the right time that will be there to support her and her children. Protect her and her children.

Thank You for revealing to her which way You want her to go in her spirit. At any time that she may fall, I thank You that You are always right there to pick her up. Help her to forgive herself and others who may offend her. I thank You for the plans that You have for her bright future.

Whatever her life purpose or destiny is, reveal it to her spirit. Confirm it with two or three witnesses. I thank You that every good work that You begin in her You will complete it. I thank You for opening the eyes of her spirit so that by faith she will see herself and others like You do. All these things I ask in Jesus' name. Amen.

Heart Vision

I know this exercise is not easy, but it needs to be done so that you can move forward. Close your eyes and look with your heart to see who you need to forgive and what they have done that you need to forgive. When you open your eyes, write in your journal what you saw.

Answer these questions in your journal:

1. Are you ready to make a decision to change your life? Why or why not?
2. Do you need resources that can help you during this transition?
3. Is there anything that you need to forgive yourself for? If so, What?
4. Do you know what your life purpose is? If so, What?

Shining Your Light

In this chapter, we talked about your being forgiven and how your ability to forgive yourself and others frees you up to fulfill your destiny.

In your journal, write four things that you can do this week to let your light shine and put your heart vision into motion.

Write these questions in your journal:

1. Are you going to make a decision to forgive and release your right to hold a grudge for those in your "Heart Vision" exercise, including yourself?

2. What resources in appendix B can you contact to help you in your transition?

3. If you don't know your life purpose, will you commit to reading *A Purpose- Driven Life* by Rick Warren?

4. If you do know your life purpose that will in some way help others, what step or steps can you take to make it happen?

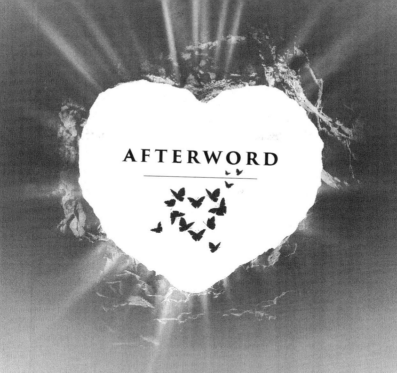

My Life Today through God's Grace

There is a song that comes to mind when I think of my life. It is the Clark Sister's song called, "I'm Looking for a Miracle." Let me give you the lyrics:

I'm looking for a miracle,
I expect the impossible,
I feel the intangible and
I see the invisible.

Bridge:
The sky is the limit
To what I can have.

Just believe and receive it,
God will perform it today,
Hey, Hey, Hey,
Just believe and receive it,
God will perform it today.

Vamp:
I expect a miracle every day,
God will make a way out of no way.

I think of this song because for many years in my first marriage, I looked for God to supernaturally work a miracle in my life. I expected it every day.

The problem was that I was not ready to receive the opportunities that God was already providing for me to take advantage of all along. I did not use my God-given authority of making choices with my free will.

God gives you plenty of opportunities. But if you don't take advantage of them, you end up missing the miracles that God has in store for you. It was not until I made the choice to move out of harm's way and get out of a destructive marriage that I was able to receive the miracle that God had in store for me.

I still believe in miracles. When I look at my life today compared to where I was in my previous marriage, it is nothing short of a miracle. My life is so different now. It is like night and day.

MY CHILDREN TODAY

Today, my children are well-adjusted, confident, and secure adults. Because I left the chaos of abuse, they now know what a peaceful home feels and looks like. They know what it's like to see love and respect modeled in front of them.

My daughter expects to be valued. She has a nursing career and aspires to be a nurse practitioner. She is now married, and I am enjoying my first granddaughter. My son told me that he wants to build up instead of tear down his home one day. He is passionately pursuing a career as a family psychologist so that he can provide therapy plans for families that struggle with the very challenges that he personally lived through.

MY WORK PLACE TODAY

While married to my ex-husband, I worked for other corporations and for other doctors. I had to leave six jobs as a professional optometrist as a direct result of my destructive marriage. I was never stable in my career.

Today, I am writing history as a female, African American entrepreneur who owns what may be the oldest, now state-of-the-art medical optical and optometric practice in Mississippi. Odom's Optical has been a staple in the eye-care community in Mississippi for more than seventy years. It was established in 1947.

I am blessed to be able to work every weekday with an experienced staff of ten professionals who have a passion to serve people from small children to geriatric residents at nursing homes that we visit and serve.

My favorite time of the month is when I invite a guest from the community to our office to give our staff a devotion before we eat lunch together. It is totally voluntary to come, and our staff is provided an opportunity to be refreshed, inspired, and grow in their faith in a safe place at work. We call this time of fellowship Faith at Work. It is inspired by what my godmother, Ms. Willa, does at her job in Montgomery.

MY MARRIAGE TODAY

Each night when I get home from work and on the weekends, I am happy to be at home to spend time with my new, loving husband. Thank God, there is no abuse. My home is just like the scripture that I confessed for years. Remember I mentioned Isaiah 32:18 before? God promises His people quiet and peaceful dwelling places. All of the prayers for my marriage that I had prayed for years, God has now answered. I was praying for the right relationship but for the wrong husband for me.

The Word of God tells me that I am wonderfully made, and my husband today looks into my eyes and tells me every day that he loves me and how beautiful I am. Instead of constantly taking from me, he constantly is giving to me, be it a kind word, a nod of reassurance, a tender touch, or a sweet kiss.

I love to hear his voice on the phone. Before he ends his calls, he always asks me, "Do you need anything?" We always share financial family obligations, but he ends up doing more than me. He tells me, "Thank you for the opportunity," when he pays for me to get my hair and nails done.

He gives me the most elaborate flower arrangements for holidays, birthdays, and just because days. We have lunch dates almost every day. And he proves that chivalry still exists. He holds my hand, gets the door, and pulls out my chair. We pray together every day. I know that my marriage is honoring Christ because of the fruit that it bears. My marriage truly glorifies God. This is my miracle.

MY CHURCH LIFE TODAY

In my previous marriage, my church life and my home life were polar opposites. Now my church life and my home life mirror each other. I was always active in church. The difference now is that I don't have to pretend that everything is okay with me and my family. What everyone sees is genuine and authentic. My married life is an open book. God's grace and mercy are evident and real in my life to inspire others.

My husband and I serve together as lay leaders at our church. This means that we have the honor of representing the members of our church at district meetings. We are liaisons between the congregation and the pastor to relay concerns and suggestions. We serve on different church committees.

We are blessed to have the opportunity to bring the message during the church service once a year as lay leaders. We are given the opportunity to "MC" some of the church services as worship leaders. We also get to teach New Believers' classes and lead a discipleship small group together.

MY EX-HUSBAND TODAY

I am happy to say that my ex-husband is working consistently in a professional career. He has remarried and has a blended family. Because he lives in another state, I don't see him often. Over the years, he has reached out to build relationships with our adult children.

Our paths cross at events where we celebrate our children.

These events have included their graduations, our daughter's wedding, and the birth of our beautiful granddaughter.

At first at these events, I would avoid him like the plague. But as time passed, and I moved through the process of forgiveness, and as members of my support group "prayed my strength in the Lord," I was able to release more grace and mercy to him, which has allowed me to feel okay when I'm around him.

YOUR MIRACLE TO LOOK FOR

What miracle are you looking for in your marriage? What's your choice? You may not make any choices because you are afraid of making the wrong decision.

Well, by not making a decision at all, you are essentially making a decision to stay where you are. Your miracle won't come. That was me! You must use your authority as a believer to use your free will and make a choice to choose your best life for yourself and your children today.

If you believe in the GPS system of the Holy Spirit, He will guide you. Do not be afraid to get into motion. As long as your heart is leading you to do it, your decision is in line with the Word of God, you have listened for God's answer in prayer, and considered godly counsel, God is waiting on you to get out of "park" and into "drive." Take your foot off the brake and put it on the gas!

Understand that God is ultimately in control. According to Jeremiah 29:11, He knows the plans that He has for your life. They are not there to harm you but to do good for you so that you can have a bright future. Have a grateful heart that is content and full of thanksgiving. Understand that if you do temporarily make a wrong turn, it is just a detour.

When you continually acknowledge and recognize Him, He will direct you how to get back on your path that He intended for you as you keep moving toward your promises and miracle.

Appendix A

EMOTIONAL ABUSE TEST[*]

Do you...

1. feel afraid of your partner much of the time?
2. avoid certain topics out of fear of angering your partner?
3. feel that you can't do anything right for your partner?
4. believe that you deserve to be hurt or mistreated?
5. wonder if you're the one who is crazy?
6. feel emotionally numb or helpless?

Does your partner...

1. humiliate or yell at you?
2. criticize you and put you down?
3. treat you so badly that you're embarrassed for your friends or family to see?
4. ignore or put down your opinions or accomplishments?
5. blame you for their own abusive behavior?
6. see you as property or a sex object rather than a person?
7. have a bad and unpredictable temper?

---

[*] Emotional abuse test adapted from *Domestic Abuse and Violence* by HealthGuide.org.

8.   hurt you or threaten to hurt or kill you?

9.   threaten to take your children away or harm them?

10. threaten to commit suicide if you leave?

11. force you to have sex?

12. destroy your belongings?

13. act excessively jealous and possessive?

14. control where you go or what you do?

15. keep you from seeing your friends or family?

16. limit your access to money, the phone, or the car?

17. constantly check up on you?

EMOTIONAL ABUSE TEST SCORING

The more questions you answered yes to in this emotional abuse quiz, the more likely it is that you are in an abusive relationship.

If you feel you are in an abusive relationship, reach out. No one deserves to be emotionally abused by another person no matter what the circumstances. Remember that you are not alone and there are people available to help you.

To get help for emotional abuse:

- Call the National Domestic Violence Hotline 1-800-799-7233 (SAFE).
- Go to www.womanslaw.org to find state and national help.
- Contact your local police or call 911 if you feel you are in immediate danger.
- Contact a child and family welfare agency.
- Talk to your doctor or other health professionals.

REFERENCE

Tracy, N. (2012, July 24). *Emotional Abuse Test: Am I Emotionally Abused?* HealthyPlace. Retrieved on 2019, August 31 from https://www.healthyplace.com/abuse/ emotional-psychological-abuse/emotioal-abuse-test-am-i -emotionally-abused.

Appendix B

Resources for Victims and Survivors of Domestic Violence

NATIONAL CRISIS ORGANIZATIONS AND ASSISTANCE

National Coalition against Domestic Violence

1-303-839-1852
www.ncadv.org

The National Domestic Violence Hotline

1-800-799-7233 (SAFE)
www.ndvh.org
(They can help you develop a safety plan.)

National Dating Abuse Helpline

1-866-331-9474
www.loveisrespect.org

National Child Abuse Hotline/Childhelp

1-800-4-A-CHILD (1-800-422-4453)
www.childhelp.org

National Sexual Assault Hotline

1-800-656-4673 (HOPE)
www.rainn.org

National Suicide Prevention Lifeline

1-800-273-8255 (TALK)
www.suicidepreventionlifeline.org

National Center for Victims of Crime

1-202-467-8700
www.victimsofcrime.org

National Human Trafficking Resource Center/Polaris Project

Call: 1-888-373-7888 | Text: HELP to BeFree (233733)
www.polarisproject.org

National Network for Immigrant and Refugee Rights

1-510-465-1984
www.nnirr.org

National Coalition for the Homeless

1-202-737-6444
www.nationalhomeless.org

National Resource Center on Domestic Violence

1-800-537-2238

www.nrcdv.org and www.vawnet.org

Futures Without Violence: The National Health Resource Center on Domestic Violence

1-888-792-2873

www.futureswithoutviolence.org

National Center on Domestic Violence, Trauma & Mental Health

1-312-726-7020 ext. 2011

www.nationalcenterdvtraumamh.org

CHILDREN

Childhelp USA/National Child Abuse Hotline

1-800-422-4453

www.childhelpusa.org

Children's Defense Fund

202-628-8787

www.childrensdefense.org

Child Welfare League of America

202-638-2952

www.cwla.org

National Council on Juvenile and Family Court Judges

Child Protection and Custody/Resource Center on Domestic Violence

1-800-527-3233
www.ncjfcj.org

Center for Judicial Excellence

info@centerforjudicialexcellence.org
www.centerforjudicialexcellence.org

TEENS

Love Is Respect

Hotline: 1-866-331-9474
www.loveisrespect.org

Break the Cycle

202-824-0707
www.breakthecycle.org

College Campus Safety Guide

https://www.bestcolleges.com/resources/
campus-safety-guide/
https://www.bestvalueschools.org/
college-campus-safety-guide/

DIFFERENTLY ABLED

Domestic Violence Initiative

(303) 839-5510/ (877) 839-5510
www.dviforwomen.org

Deaf Abused Women's Network (DAWN)

Email: Hotline@deafdawn.org

VP: 202-559-5366

www.deafdawn.org

WOMEN OF COLOR

Women of Color Network

1-800-537-2238

www.wocninc.org

INCITE! Women of Color Against Violence

incite.natl@gmail.com

www.incite-national.org

LATINA/LATINO

Casa de Esperanza

Linea de crisis 24-horas/24-hour crisis line

1-651-772-1611

www.casadeesperanza.org

National Latin@ Network for Healthy Families and Communities

1-651-646-5553

www.nationallatinonetwork.org

IMMIGRANT

The National Immigrant Women's Advocacy Project

(202) 274-4457

http://www.niwap.org/

INDIGENOUS WOMEN

National Indigenous Women's Resource Center

855-649-7299

www.niwrc.org

Indigenous Women's Network

1-512-258-3880

www.indigenouswomen.org

ASIAN/PACIFIC ISLANDER

Asian and Pacific Islander Institute on Domestic Violence

1-415-954-9988

www.apiidv.org

Committee Against Anti-Asian Violence (CAAAV)

1-212- 473-6485

www.caaav.org

Manavi

1-732-435-1414

www.manavi.org

AFRICAN AMERICAN

Institute on Domestic Violence in the African American Community

1-877-643-8222

www.dvinstitute.org

The Black Church and Domestic Violence Institute

1-770-909-0715

www.bcdvi.org

ABUSE IN LATER LIFE

National Clearinghouse on Abuse in Later Life

1-608-255-0539

www.ncall.us

National Center for Elder Abuse

1-855-500-3537

www.aginginplace.org

MEN

National Organization for Men against Sexism (NOMAS)

1-720-466-3882

www.nomas.org

A Call to Men

1-917-922-6738

www.acalltomen.org

Men Can Stop Rape

1-202-265-6530

www.mencanstoprape.org

Men Stopping Violence

1-866-717-9317

www.menstoppingviolence.org

LEGAL

Battered Women's Justice Project
1-800-903-0111
www.bwjp.org

Legal Momentum
1-212-925-6635
www.legalmomentum.org

Womenslaw.org
www.womenslaw.org

National Clearinghouse for the Defense of Battered Women
1-800-903-0111 x 3
www.ncdbw.org

Legal Network for Gender Equity
nwlc.org/join-the-legal-network/

RESOURCES FOR THOSE WORKING WITH VICTIMS AND SURVIVORS OF DOMESTIC VIOLENCE

HELPFUL BRIEFS AND PAPERS

- From Responding to Intimate Violence in Relationship Programs (RIViR)
- The US Department of Health and Services – Administration of Children and Families

- https://www.acf.hhs.gov/sites/default/files/opre/rivir_paper_2_current_approaches_4_6_16_clean_psg_b508_2.pdf
- https://www.acf.hhs.gov/sites/default/files/opre/rivir_paper_1_prevalence_3_29_16_complete_b508.pdf

OTHER RESOURCES

Financial Assistance for Mothers

Give Her Wings
www.giveherwings.com

PLANNING

Family Renewal Shelter

1-253-475-9010
1-888-550-3915
www.domesticviolencehelp.com
(A Christian resource that helps with crisis and safety planning.)

Safety Planning Example

www.theraveproject.com/index.php/resource_content/personalized_safety_plan
www.overcomingpowerlessness.com/safety_plan.htm.

PROFESSIONAL CHRISTIAN COUNSELORS
DOMESTIC VIOLENCE SPECIALISTS

Focus on the Family Counselors

1-800-232-6459

http://family.custhelp.com/app/home (find a counselor)

American Association of Christian Counselors

https://www.aacc.net/

Appendix C

Prayers

PRAYER OF SALVATION

If you want to be forgiven by God and know that you are a part of His family, you can say a simple prayer like this out loud so that you can hear yourself praying to Him:

"Father God, I believe that Jesus Christ is the Son of God. I believe that Jesus died on the cross to pay the penalty for my sins. I believe that He arose from the dead and is alive today. Please forgive me for my sins. Lord Jesus, come into my life right now. Come into my heart now and be my Lord and Savior.

I believe in my heart and confess with my mouth that Jesus Christ is right now my personal Lord and Savior. Thank you, God, that I am right now born again! Amen."

As soon as you choose to believe in God and sincerely say this prayer aloud, He gives you the power of the Holy Spirit that comes to live in your heart who enables you to fulfill the purpose that He has planned for your life. The Holy Spirit gives you the character traits of God, called the fruit of the Spirit, which I mentioned in chapter 1. He gives you the power to forgive yourself and others so that your heart can heal. Next, ask Him to give you the power of the Holy Spirit to come upon you to be a bold witness for Christ.

Congratulations! I rejoice with you on today being your spiritual birthday! Now find a church that is preaching the Word of God in such a way that you can grow and develop. Let the pastor know that you just received Christ into your heart. Ask for any resources that they may have to assist you on your new journey with God.

Continually watch whom you stay in fellowship with. Seek the company of other believers whom you can gain wisdom from and who can encourage you. Set aside a few minutes each day to pray, listen for God's voice, and read the Bible. Get a devotional app for your phone or a book for new believers.

PRAYER OF REDEDICATION

If you have already asked Jesus to come into your heart, but your relationship with Him is not close anymore, and you would like to be in closer fellowship with Him, you can say a simple prayer like this:

"Father God, I admit that there have been times that I've chosen to do things my way instead of Yours. Please forgive me for (say the things that you have missed the mark on). I thank You, Jesus, for Your blood that washes away my sins and that You are praying for me on my behalf to Father God right now. I thank You, God for Your everlasting love and that You are faithful and just and that You forgive me for everything that I have done that is not right in Your sight. I

thank You for the power to forgive myself. I thank You that today, I am the righteousness of God in Christ Jesus. In Jesus' name. Amen."

Hallelujah! I praise God for new beginnings. I have definitely messed up and fell short of what brings glory to God at times in my life. But let me say this: Even though God gives us grace and mercy when we sin, this does not give us free license to continually and willfully sin and take advantage of His provisions. What you do continually reveals your true character. We cannot fool Him. He knows the intentions of our hearts. God is a merciful God. But He is also a God of justice. We will all have to stand before his judgment seat and account for what we have done in our bodies.

Even when you are a child of God, you still will mess up because you are human. But as His child, you are going to want to get it straight because you love your Father God very much. You have to be willing to receive God's grace for yourself.

Do not allow the devil to beat you up in your mind. The Word of God says the devil is the "accuser" of God's children. You continue to agree with the devil if you keep blaming yourself for your mistakes. Then the devil is victorious with his mission to keep you defeated. Don't play into his tactics. Just thank God for His unmerited mercy and grace. Live in the freedom of His forgiveness that He willingly provides for you.

REFERENCE SCRIPTURES

But what does scripture say? "The word is near you; it is in your mouth and in your heart," that is, the message concerning faith that we proclaim: "If you declare with your mouth, 'Jesus is Lord,' and believe in your heart that God raised Him from the dead, you will be saved. For it is with your heart that you believe and are justified, and it is with your mouth that you profess your faith and are saved." Romans 10:8-10 (NIV)

"But you will receive power when the Holy Spirit comes upon you. And you will be my witnesses." Acts 1:8a (NLT)

"If we confess our sins, He is faithful and just to forgive us our sins, and to cleanse us from all unrighteousness." 1 John 1:9 (KJV)

"My dear children, I write this to you that your will not sin. But if anybody does sin, we have an advocate with the Father–Jesus Christ, the Righteous one." 1 John 2:1 (NIV)

"Therefore, since we have a great high priest who has ascended into heaven, Jesus the Son of God, let us hold firmly to the faith we profess. For we do not have a high priest who is unable to empathize with our weaknesses, but we have one who has been tempted in every way, just as we are–yet he did not sin. Let us then approach God's throne of grace with confidence, so that we may receive mercy and find grace to help us in our time of need." Hebrews 4:14-16 (NIV)

"Who then will condemn us? No one—for Christ Jesus died for us and was raised to life for us, and he is sitting in the place of honor at God's right hand, pleading for us." Romans 8:34 (NLT)

"Then I heard a loud voice saying in heaven, 'Now salvation, and strength, and the kingdom of our God, and the power of His Christ have come, for the accuser of our brethren, who accused them before our God day and night, has been cast down (from heaven).'" Revelations 12:10 (NKJV)

"God made him who had no sin to be sin for us, so that in him we might become the righteousness of God." 2 Corinthians 5:21 (NIV)

"We are made right with God (the righteousness of God) by placing our faith in Jesus Christ. And this is true for everyone who believes, no matter who we are." Romans 3:22 (NLT)

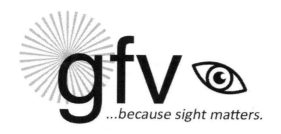

...because sight matters.

GIVE THE GIFT OF SIGHT

One dollar is donated to charity for every copy of *Heart Vision* that is sold. This charitable organization is **Great Faith Vision**.

Great Faith Vision needs your help!

They need *your help* to further their mission to provide both **physical and spiritual vision** by spreading the Good News of the Gospel and providing eye care services, eyeglasses, and medical care (including surgery and medications) to those without access or without the means to afford these services in the USA and around the world.

Great Faith Vision partners with host pastors, missionaries, and community organizations, including shelters, to open doors to the Gospel by providing these services to their communities.

Great Faith Vision is dependent on volunteers, prayers, and financial support of people like you who share their passion.

To give on-line go to:
www.gfv.org

GFV is an all-volunteer, faith based, 501 (c) 3 tax exempt nonprofit. All donations to this charity are tax deductible.

Thank you

About the Author

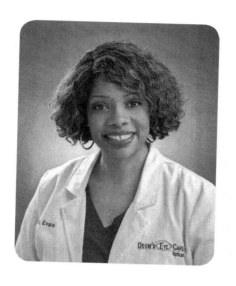

DR. DELLIA EVANS is a well-respected optometrist who has helped over 250,000 patients to improve their vision for over 25 years. Dr. Dellia helps people to see more clearly both physically and spiritually. She earned a B.A. Cum Laude from the University of Mississippi and a Doctor of Optometry degree from The University of Alabama at Birmingham. A resident of Jackson, Mississippi, she is happily re-married and has two adult children and one granddaughter.